For
Sandy & Gene
with love —

Tali
May 2001.

Pharmacracy

Pharmacracy

MEDICINE AND POLITICS
IN AMERICA

Thomas Szasz

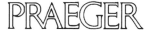 PRAEGER

Westport, Connecticut
London

Library of Congress Cataloging-in-Publication Data

Szasz, Thomas Stephen, 1920–
 Pharmacracy : medicine and politics in America / Thomas Szasz.
  p. cm.
 Includes bibliographical references and index.
 ISBN 0–275–97196–1 (alk. paper)
 1. Social medicine—United States—Miscellanea. 2. Medical care—Political
aspects—United States. 3. Medical ethics—United States. I. Title.
RA418.3.U6S936 2001
362.1'0973—dc21   00–064948

British Library Cataloguing in Publication Data is available.

Library of Congress Catalog Card Number: 00–064948
ISBN: 0–275–97196–1

First published in 2001

Praeger Publishers, 88 Post Road West, Westport, CT 06881
An imprint of Greenwood Publishing Group, Inc.
www.praeger.com

Printed in the United States of America

The paper used in this book complies with the
Permanent Paper Standard issued by the National
Information Standards Organization (Z39.48–1984).

10 9 8 7 6 5 4 3 2 1

For George,
my teacher, my friend, my brother,
with gratitude and love

The species of oppression by which democratic nations are menaced is unlike anything that ever before existed in the world; our contemporaries will find no prototype of it in their memories. I seek in vain for an expression that will accurately convey the whole of the idea I have formed of it; the old words *despotism* and *tyranny* are inappropriate: the thing itself is new. . . . The first thing that strikes the observer is an innumerable multitude of men, all equal and alike, incessantly endeavoring to procure their petty and paltry pleasures with which they glut their lives. . . . Above this race of men stands an immense and tutelary power, which takes upon itself alone to secure their gratifications and to watch over their fate. The power is absolute, minute, regular, provident, and mild. It would be like the authority of a parent if, like that authority, its object was to prepare men for manhood; but it seeks, on the contrary, to keep them in perpetual childhood. . . . For their happiness such a government willingly labors . . . provides for their security . . . facilitates their pleasures, manages their principal concerns . . . what remains, but to spare them all the care of thinking and all the trouble of living?

Alexis de Tocqueville (1805–1859)
A. de Tocqueville, *Democracy in America*, vol. 2, p. 336.

CONTENTS

Contents

PREFACE

Neither must we suppose that any one of the citizens belongs to himself, for they all belong to the state, and are each of them a part of the state, and the care of each part is inseparable from the care of the whole.

Aristotle[1]

Physicians, politicians, public policy experts, people in nearly every walk of life spend a great deal of time and energy debating what is and what is not a disease or a treatment. Although these questions appear to be about phenomena or facts, they are, more often than not, about policies or strategies. Formerly, we approved and disapproved, permitted and prohibited various behaviors because they were virtuous or wicked, legal or illegal. Now, we do so because they are deemed healthy or sick, therapeutic or pathogenic. Hence the seemingly unappeasable thirst to medicalize, pathologize, and therapeutize all manner of *behaviors* manifesting as personal or social *problems*.

The upshot is that we tend to substitute ostensibly medical criteria for explicitly moral criteria for judging character and personal conduct and use pseudomedical arguments to justify the expansion and exercise of state power. How has this transformation come about, and why do we embrace it as if it were medical, moral, and political progress?

In the ancient world, as the epigraph by Aristotle illustrates, the individual was not a person unless he was a part of the *polis*; the personal and the political were intimately interrelated. Today, under American constitutional principles, the personal and the political are distinct spheres, the desires of individuals are often in conflict with the needs of the group or the nation or the state, and this conflict is often obscured by invalidating the individual's desires as the "symptoms of illness."

If the welfare of the individual and the welfare of the collective are considered to coincide, then the ill health or ill conduct of each endangers that of the other. In the absence of clear separation between the personal and the political, the private and the public, there can be no separation between private health and public health. The personal then becomes political and politics becomes, intrinsically, "therapeutic." (Henceforth, I shall avoid placing words like "medical" and "therapy" between scare quotes to indicate their metaphorical or ironic use and let the context clarify my meaning.)

The Reformation and the Enlightenment created a sharp division between the personal and the political, perhaps nowhere more so than in the newly founded American republic. Yet, the more public policy recognizes and respects this division, the more politically divisive become the conflicts between the wants of the person and the needs of the polity. "A man may not always eat and drink what is good for him," said George Santayana (1863–1952), the great American philosopher, "but it is better for him and less ignominious to die of the gout freely than to have a censor officially appointed over his diet, who after all could not render him immortal."[2] Gilbert K. Chesterton (1874–1936), a conservative Catholic journalist and social critic, took for granted that "the free man owns himself. He can damage himself with either eating or drinking; he can ruin himself with gambling. If he does he is certainly a damn fool, and he might possibly be a damned soul; but if he may not, he is not a free man any more than a dog."[3]

Today, hardly any right-thinking person holds these beliefs. Collectivists and totalitarians dream of the brotherhood of man—protecting one another and the fatherland from enemies within and without. Individualists and libertarians long to be left alone by the state—although, in their hearts, too, there often lurks the temptation to enlist its protection when certain dangers threaten. How are we to reconcile these seemingly irreconcilable aspirations? The modern mind has seized on the ideas of disease and treatment as offering common ground. Disease often threatens, and treatment often benefits, individuals and groups alike. Saving people from disease, like saving their souls, is a good that no one (in his right mind) could have reason to reject. In the words of former Surgeon General C. Everett Koop: "The government has a perfect right to influence *behavior* to the best of its ability if it is for the welfare of the individual and the community as a whole."[4] That is a dangerous opinion, the more so because ever fewer people realize that it is dangerous.

With victory in World War II and the Cold War, the United States bestrides the world like no power has since the Roman Empire. Because politics, by definition, entails the exercise of power, and because the most elementary exercise of power is waging war, American hegemony presents a problem: there is no literal enemy to subdue. Yet, just as the metabolism of the body anatomic requires nutrients, so the metabolism of the body politic requires enemies or, at least, scapegoats. In a tacit compact, rulers and ruled unite to create enemies by alienating parts of their own nation or aspects of human nature itself: "They" are "diseases," caused by microbes, genes, chemicals out of balance, economic exploitation, or abusive parents—and "they" are attacking "us." They are wicked. We are virtuous.

The experts tell us that we eat too much, drink too much, smoke too much, gamble too much, take too many drugs; that we behave irresponsibly with respect to sex, marriage, procreation, exercise, and health care; that we commit too many murders and suicides, too many assaults, thefts, and rapes; and that all these things are not really our own doings but the manifestations of maladies. In the past, politicians seized power by declaring national emergencies. Now they do so by declaring public health emergencies. Alcoholism, obesity, suicide, and violence, they say, are killing Americans. Individuals are not responsible for eating or drinking too much, for killing themselves or others. The rejection of personal responsibility for one behavior after another—each deliberate act transformed into a "no-fault disease"—drives the politics of therapy. The government declares war on drugs, cancer, heart disease, obesity, mental illness, poverty, racism, sexism, suicide, and violence. However, drug addicts refuse to abstain from drugs, the obese overeat, the mentally sick reject being treated as patients, and the poor refuse to adopt the habits of the rich. Coping with these and other "health emergencies" requires enlarging the scope and coercive powers of medicine as an arm of the state.

In the long run, neither exaggerating the claims or rights of the individual nor exaggerating the obligations and beneficence of the state serves the cause of expanding liberty under law. We live in societies more complex than ever and are dependent on one another more, and more anonymously, than ever. No person can be free without shouldering his responsibilities, and no society can endure without penalizing irresponsible behavior. Liberty is undermined by the irresponsible individual and is destroyed by tyrannical government.

Biologically, we are animals and, as such, we are predators or prey or both. To avoid becoming prey, we live in groups—families, tribes, states—whose rules regulate our conduct. The concept of the state as guardian—parent, sovereign, or night watchman, protecting members of the group from enemies without and within—is basic to Western political philosophy. However, because of man's predatory nature—*homo homini lupus* ("man is a wolf to man"), as the Romans put it—this idea is intrinsically self-contradictory. What is there to prevent the guardians from yielding to the temptation to prey on the people they are supposed to protect? We may think of political philosophy as beginning when the Roman poet and satirist Juvenal (c. 60–140) posed the classic question: "*Quis custodiet ipsos custodes?*" "Who shall guard the guardians?"

Throughout history, most people have preferred to ignore this challenge. For a very long time, people sought comfort in guardians whose goodness was guaranteed by God, which let them place their trust in rulers whom they regarded as deputies of a deity, exemplified by the divine rule of popes and Christian sovereigns. The founders of the United States formed a different plan for protecting the American people from their own protectors. They and their compatriots regarded themselves as competent and responsible adults. Thus, the American Revolution was, in effect, a revolt of the grown child against his father intent on keeping him in tutelage: it was a demand for the self-government and self-responsibility that befits a dignified person, not for more largesse for a ward victimized by his dependence. This is what gave the Founders the strength to resist the temptation to replace one paternal government with another. Instead, they sought to create a nonpaternal government and they proceeded to construct one.

Like a fearful child dreaming of a fairy godmother, the puerile mind dreams of the trustworthy ruler. Liberated from that delusion, the mature mind recognizes not only that power corrupts but also that those who seek power tend to be corrupt, and hence distrusts all rulers. Rulers ought to be watched with suspicion, not worshiped. Thus, the Founders endeavored to avoid the danger of despotic government by limiting its scope—delegating powers to states composing a confederation of independent political units—and by creating a government of divided powers—one branch checking and balancing the powers of the others. Although never fully realized, that, at least in theory, was the vision that characterized American polity from 1787 until 1861.

Today, that vision is a thing of a past existentially more distant from us than ancient Rome was from the Founders. The Founders understood that the greatest danger to man is other men, especially when they are out to protect him from himself. Forgetting that maxim, modern man thirsted for powerful rulers to protect him and, in the twentieth century, he found just what he was looking for: These "strong men" managed to kill more people, including their own, than have all past rulers combined.

What do we now fear the most? The answer, issuing from the most respected sources, is loud and clear: responsibility for our own behavior. The dominant ethic rests on two premises: (1) We are responsible only for our good deeds; (2) our bad deeds are diseases or the products of diseases for which we are not responsible. This doctrine tells us that we can no more combat alcoholism and panic disorder with will power than we can amebiasis and parkinsonism. Only treatment can remedy such problems. Our duty is to pay more taxes, to enable government scientists to discover cures for these diseases, and to recognize that we are ill and place ourselves in the care of health care agents of the state, to begin the lifelong process of recovery. "I would hopefully be a good role model. I'm in recovery," declares Cindy McCain, wife of Senator and former presidential hopeful John McCain (R-Az).[5] Mrs. McCain had used controlled substances that she had stolen while she worked as a member of a "charity she had set up to send medical relief to the Third World."[6] The one thing we must not do is assume that how we live is our own business and responsibility. This package is now usually sold under the label of promoting "patient autonomy," a term that, as I showed elsewhere, is now an integral part of the semantics of social control through medicine.[7]

While awaiting medical research to solve the riddle of the biological roots of problematic behaviors conceptualized as diseases and provide a cure for them, people must, however, cope with the personal and social problems they face. Cope with them they do, as predators are predisposed to, by waging literal wars on people allegedly suffering from the metaphorical plagues of drugs, racism, violence, and human nature itself. The delusionary goal of an America free of drugs, free of disease, free of strife, suicide, and violence—of death itself—justifies these wars waged by a tacit agreement between a populace eager to reject responsibility for self-discipline and its political representatives eagerly pandering to that longing. How? By declaring that human problems are diseases that medicine will soon conquer, just as it has conquered polio and smallpox. Thus, the boundaries of medicine expand until they encompass all human aspirations and actions.

Comforted by the delusionary concept of "no-fault disease," the illness inflation set in motion by the medicalization of (mis)behavior accelerates and, in turn, intensifies the tendency to reject responsibility for (mis)behavior. We are loath to use the criminal laws to control genuine criminals, that is, people who deprive others of life, liberty, or property. We are unwilling to control our children, who, in turn, are unwilling or unable to control their own behavior. Judges sentence criminals to "treatment programs," and school authorities—aided and abetted by physicians, psychologists, and parents—manage unruly children with "prescription drugs" and lectures about our national struggle for a "drug-free America." Truly, we have become Santayana's "fanatics" who, after losing sight of their goal, redouble their effort.

Actually, we Americans are now healthier than we have ever been and live longer than we have ever lived. Why, then, do we perceive our existential problems in medical terms and seek their solution in a tyranny exercised by therapeutic tribunes? Why should a healthy people dread disease so much? Although the fear may seem paradoxical, there is logic in it.

In 1776, Americans enjoyed more political freedom than they ever did as Englishmen or colonists. That is precisely why they valued liberty and were zealous in guarding it against tyrannical rulers. It is the free and the rich, not the enslaved and the poor, who worry about losing their liberty and their money and seek to protect themselves from those dangers. It is the healthy, not the sick, who worry about losing their health and seek to protect themselves from that danger. We are medically richer than people have ever been. We have gained more control over real diseases than we would have dreamed possible a hundred years ago. It is precisely these advances that have encouraged extending the idiom, imagery, and technology of medicine to other areas of human concern, transforming all sorts of human problems into "diseases," and the rule of law into the rule of medicine, in a word, "pharmacracy."[8]

A brief remark about this term is in order here. The Greek term *pharmakon*—a so-called primal word, possessing antithetical meanings—meant both drug and poison. The term *pharmakos* referred to a ceremonially sacrificed scapegoat, whose death purified and thus cured/saved the community. In 1976, in *Ceremonial Chemistry*, I wrote: "Inasmuch as we have words to describe medicine as a healing art, but have none to describe it as a method of social control or political rule, we must first give it a name. I propose that we call it *pharmacracy*, from the Greek roots *pharmakon*, for 'medicine' or 'drug,' and *kratein,* for 'to rule' or 'to control.' . . . As theocracy is rule by God or priests, and democracy is rule by the people or the majority, so pharmacracy is rule by medicine or physicians."[9] In a theocracy, people perceive all manner of human problems as religious in nature, susceptible to religious remedies; similarly, in a pharmacracy people perceive all manner of human problems as medical in nature, susceptible to medical remedies. Specifically, I shall use the term "pharmacratic controls" to refer to social sanctions exercised by bureaucratic health-care regulations, enforced by health-care personnel, such as alcohol treatment and other addiction programs, school psychology, suicide prevention, and the mandatory reporting of personal (mis)behavior as part of the duties of physicians and other health-care personnel.

My aim in this book is to show that the effort to medicalize life is not only cognitively ill-conceived, it is also politically perilous. Conflict is intrinsic to human existence. Regulating disagreements as if they were diseases is a recipe for forfeiting liberty in pursuit of an illusory therapeutic paradise on earth.

ACKNOWLEDGMENTS

I am most grateful to my brother George, daughter Margot Peters, son-in-law Steve Peters, and my friends Alice Michtom, Robert Schneebeli, and Roger Yanow for their extensive corrections, comments, criticisms, and suggestions. This acknowledgment does not do justice to their contribution, let alone their patient labors. I also cannot do justice to acknowledging the generous help of Peter Uva, librarian at the State University of New York Upstate Medical University, with this book and with many others in the past. Finally, I wish to thank the Greenwood Publishing Group for producing books by an author who—paraphrasing Samuel Butler—never writes on any subject unless he believes the opinion of those who have the ear of the public to be mistaken, and this involves, as a necessary consequence, that every book he writes runs counter to the men who are in possession of the field.[1]

ABBREVIATIONS

ADHD	attention deficit hyperactivity disorder
AIDS	acquired immune deficiency syndrome
AMA	American Medical Association
APA	American Psychiatric Association
AWDA	Americans with Disabilities Act
DEA	drug enforcement agency
DOT	directly observed therapy
DRG	diagnosis-related group
DSM	*Diagnostic and Statistical Manual of Mental Disorders* (of the APA)
HMO	health maintenance organization
ICD	International Classification of Diseases
NHS	National Health Service (UK)
NIDA	National Institute of Drug Abuse
NIH	National Institutes of Health
NIMH	National Institute of Mental Health
PTSD	posttraumatic stress disorder
S.S.R.I.	selective serotonin reuptake inhibitor
SUNY	State University of New York

Abbreviations

VIP	very important person
VUP	very unimportant person
WHO	World Health Organization

INTRODUCTION
What Counts as a Disease?

Vicissitudes of fashion will enforce the use of new, or extend the significa-
tion of known terms. The tropes of poetry will make hourly encroach-
ments, and the metaphorical will become the current sense . . . illiterate
writers will at one time or other, by publick infatuation, rise in renown,
who, not knowing the original import of words, will use them with collo-
quial licentiousness, confound distinction, and forget propriety.

Samuel Johnson (1775)[1]

What is a disease? What is *not* a disease? Although most people think they
know the answer, few have a clear idea of what is and what is not a disease. This
is hardly surprising. The word "disease"—and its synonyms, "ailment," "illness," "malady," "sickness"—is used in diverse ways and has a multiplicity of
meanings. In the end, people decide what is and what is not a disease by what
best suits their needs or on the basis of the hoary rule, "I know one when I see
one."

To bring order to our disorderly use of language, we distinguish between the
literal and the metaphorical uses of terms. The root meaning of the term
"honey," for example, names the substance secreted by bees. When a man calls
his wife "honey," he is speaking metaphorically. The distinction between literal
and metaphorical meaning is, of course, a matter of convention: it requires
agreement about the root meaning of the particular term. The point is that unless we assign a *discrete, limited, identifiable* meaning to a term, we cannot dis-

tinguish between its literal and metaphorical uses and cannot use the term with precision.

Our enquiry must therefore begin with a clarification of the root meaning of the term "disease." To what object or phenomenon does the term refer? Framed about particulars, there is likely to be general agreement about the answer: typhoid fever is a disease, spring fever is not. However, framed abstractly, there is likely to be disagreement. Why? Because we lack unanimity about *why we regard typhoid fever, but not spring fever, as a disease.* That is why we fruitlessly debate whether drug addiction, clinical depression, pathological gambling, social anxiety, and so forth are or are not diseases. Unless we agree on the root meaning of the term "disease," we *cannot know* what counts as a literal disease and what counts as a metaphorical disease, that is, not a true disease. Similar considerations account for the futility of debating whether abortion, euthanasia, surgical remedies for transsexualism, and many other procedures performed by physicians are or are not treatments.

Knowing the difference between the literal and metaphorical uses and meanings of words is not a special skill. It is a matter of knowing how to use language properly. In certain areas of life—religion, in particular—individuals willingly suspend their knowledge of this distinction, a sacred text becoming "literally" the word of God. I regard this as evidence of the near-universality of the understanding of the distinction between the literal and the metaphorical. Clearly, even people unfamiliar with the terms "literal" and "metaphorical" recognize the difference. Everyday speech, humor, poetry, and technical jargon all depend on enriching literal meanings with figures of speech. Some viruses attack the immune system, others attack computer programs. No one mistakes computer viruses for biological agents.

This book is, in part, an argument about what should count as a disease. How that argument is resolved affects so many aspects of everyday life that it may be no exaggeration to say it is the single most important issue in contemporary American life. "What is the good of words if they aren't important enough to quarrel over?" asked G. K. Chesterton. "Why do we choose one word more than another if there isn't any difference between them? If you called a woman a chimpanzee instead of an angel, wouldn't there be a quarrel about words? If you are not going to argue about words, what are you going to argue about?"[2] If we fail to settle the argument about what should count as a disease, or settle it on the basis of capricious, politically grounded criteria, we incapacitate ourselves from thinking clearly about what should count as health care or treatment, who should pay for it, and the many other health policy issues we now argue about.

Failure to distinguish between the literal and figurative uses of words may be due to ignorance or, when powerful human interests are at stake, may be a part of a deliberate strategy and an institutionally mandated policy. Our use of the verb "to medicalize" is instructive in this connection: the locution depends on and betrays a *tacit understanding of the limited scope of medicine, and hence of the core meaning of disease.* We speak about medicalizing suicide or violence, tacitly acknowledging that we are enlarging the scope of medicine, and we recognize the absurdity of speaking about medicalizing malaria or melanoma, tacitly acknowledging the proper sphere of medicine. Similar considerations hold for the terms "politicize" and "theologize." (*Webster's Third New International Dictionary* and the *Oxford English Dictionary* both have entries for "politicize" and "theologize," but neither has an entry for "medicalize.")

When religion reigned and church and government were united in a theological state, people perceived countless human problems as the products of divine or satanic intervention, and sought to remedy them with appropriate religious interventions, such as prayer and exorcism. When science reigns and medicine and the government are united in a therapeutic state, people perceive countless human problems as the products of diseases, and seek to remedy them with medical interventions, such as drugs and "therapy." I should note here, perhaps, that I coined the term "therapeutic state" in 1963 with deliberate irony, as a critical and dishonorific sobriquet, to denote the political union of medicine and the state, physicians playing the same sorts of ambiguous, double roles that priests played when church and state were united. The ambiguity, coercion, and paternalism intrinsic to such a role of the physician— sometimes helping the patient, sometimes harming him—is incompatible with individual dignity, liberty, responsibility, and the rule of law. I regard the therapeutic state as a type of totalitarian state, persecutions in the name of health by doctors replacing persecutions in the name of God by priests.[3] (Some writers now use the term approvingly, denoting a medicalized variant of the welfare state or an ideal, scientifically enlightened polity.)

As a science, medicine rests on and makes use of the same methods and principles as the physical sciences. One of these principles is that the observer is a person, and the object he observes is not. Chemists and physicists observe, for example, the characteristics of various elements and classify them as helium, lithium, uranium, and so forth. The classification serves the interests of the classifiers. The objects classified have no interests.

To understand the many conceptual, economic, and political problems that beset contemporary medical practice, that is, *medicine as health care,* we must distinguish between scientific medicine, whose objects of study are diseases that affect human beings, and clinical medicine, whose objects of study are persons, usually called "patients." Making this distinction does not imply that one is intellectually, morally, or practically better or more important than the other. Each enterprise has its own agenda and vocabulary.

Introduction

- The aim of scientific medicine, an enterprise barely 150 years old, is to increase our understanding of the causes and cures of conditions scientifically defined as diseases. The aim of clinical medicine, which may be said to be as old as civilization, is to help persons regarded as sick recover their health.

- The practitioner of medical science seeks to understand disease. The practitioner of clinical medicine seeks to relieve dis-ease.

- Scientific medical knowledge is indifferent to individual or collective human well-being; it may be equally useful for biological warfare and the relief of human suffering. In contrast, the *raison d'être* of clinical medicine is the welfare of the patient.

Diverse concepts of disease—ranging from the objective to the subjective, from the literal to the metaphorical, from uremia to insomnia—are now compelled to coexist, in scientific, clinical, and political medicine. Compelled by whom? By authorities in science, medicine, the media, politics, and the law, in a word, by the *Zeitgeist*. The suggestion that, say, AIDS and ADHD (acquired immune deficiency syndrome and attention deficit hyperactivity disorder) are radically different kinds of diseases—or, more precisely, that the latter is not a disease at all—is politically so incorrect that it is dismissed out of hand.

Without a solid consensus on what is a literal disease, how would we recognize a metaphorical disease if we met one?

1

MEDICINE
From Gnostic Healing to Empirical Science

For he [God] makes sore, and bindeth up: he woundeth, and his hands make whole.

Job 5:17–18

Disease: A condition of the body, or of some part or organ of the body, in which its functions are disturbed or deranged; a morbid physical condition.

Oxford English Dictionary

In the ancient world, disease was a gnostic concept, concerned with "spiritual truth," not with empirical evidence. In Biblical, Greek, and Roman accounts, disease is a holistic-theistic concept that precludes distinguishing between literal and metaphorical illnesses, between diseases of the body and diseases of the mind. There is no Latin word for our scientific concept of disease. When the Romans spoke of disease, they used the word *"morbus"*—the root of the English words "morbid" and "morbidity"—which also means disaster, fault, and vice; or the word *"malum"*—the root of such English words as "malefactor" and "malevolent"—which also means evil, harm, hardship, and punishment.[1] The King James Version of the Scriptures uses the terms "murrain," "plague," and "pestilence," instead of the term "disease." The Revised Standard Version uses "plague" throughout. Accordingly, the act of healing entailed intermingling natural and supernatural means of influence, medical and religious methods of treating the body and the mind.

In the biblical view, as the story of Job illustrates, the cause of both disease and cure is God. Vexed by Job's piety, Satan seeks God's permission to tempt Job to curse the Lord and thus demonstrate his moral imperfection. "And the Lord said unto Satan, Behold, he is in thine hand. . . . So went Satan forth from the presence of the Lord, and smote Job with sore boils from the sole of his foot unto his crown."[2] The parable demonstrates God's medical omnipotence: "Behold, happy is the man whom God correcteth. . . . *For he makes sore, and bindeth up: he woundeth, and his hands make whole.*"[3]

Ancient gnostic concepts of disease and treatment are incommensurable with their modern, materialist counterparts. In the gnostic view, both disease and treatment are the results of divine intervention—the former, punishment for sinning, the latter, reward for repentance. In the materialist view, both disease and treatment are "natural" processes—the former having many possible causes, often microbes, the latter typically cured by chemicals, often available by prescription only.

From the materialist point of view, the phenomenon of disease is, of course, older than the human race and affects all life forms. Sir Marc Armand Ruffer (1859–1917), one of the founders of paleopathology—the science of the diseases "that can be demonstrated in human and animal remains of ancient times"—observed that "wild primates suffer from many disorders, including arthritis, malaria, hernia, parasitic worms, and impacted teeth. Our ancestors presumably experienced disorders and diseases similar to those found among modern primates."[4]

Hippocratic medicine is a blend of gnostic and materialist elements. Instead of viewing disease as a discrete lesion or process, the Hippocratics saw it as a disturbance affecting the whole person through an imbalance among the four humors, blood, phlegm, black bile, and yellow bile. These humors, together with the four associated qualities—hot, cold, moist, and dry—form the microcosm of the human body and reflect the four elements—earth, air, fire, and water—that make up the macrocosm or universe. "Health is the result of the harmonious balance or blending of the four humors."[5]

I recapitulate these familiar facts to underscore that whereas the humoral model of disease is holistic, etiological, and spiritual, the pathological model of it is localized, phenomenological, and material. I do this to show that, contrary to the claims of its supporters, the modern biopsychosocial image of illness—emphasizing explanation over phenomenon and treatment over understanding—represents a regression to the prescientific conception of illness, not a progression beyond the pathological conception of it.

THE IDEA OF ILLNESS: A BRIEF HISTORY

In the ancient world, people feared and held the dead body in superstitious awe. This sentiment, deeply seated in the human mind, continues to linger in the popular imagination and forms one of the permanent sources of religion. As long as this sentiment was strong and socially sanctioned as rational, it precluded examining a dead body to study its structure and function. Doing so would have violated an unarticulated taboo, rooted in the Greeks' fear of and aversion to caducity, manifested by their idealization of the youthful, hale, whole, and healthy. This is why Hippocrates had not the faintest idea about what is inside the body, a subject into which he neither wished nor dared to inquire.

Although Aristotle studied animals and is sometimes said to be the founder of comparative anatomy, he believed that the heart is the seat of the intellect, because it beats. The anatomical fantasies of the ancients were systematized by Galen (2nd century A.D.), the most famous physician of antiquity. The Jewish, Christian, and Islamic religions catered to man's instinctive dread of the dead body by prohibiting the dissection of the corpse. For the next thousand years, physicians studied books, not bodies. The answers to the riddles of disease lay in the writings of Aristotle and Galen, not in observation and experiment. This situation lasted roughly until the Enlightenment.

How could the premodern physician, ignorant of the makeup of the body, treat diseases? The story of prescientific healing has been told many times and does not belong here. Like the quack today, the ancient healer, too, was convinced that he knew what he was doing and his customers were satisfied with his services. One of the most absurd conceits of modernity is the belief that our sick forebears were bereft of medical help. For minor maladies—such as colds or small wounds, viewed as a natural part of everyday life—they had a vast array of herbal medicines. For major maladies—such as the "plague," viewed as due to supernatural sources—they had priests, prayer, and scapegoats to sacrifice to the gods. Indeed, if diseases are perceived as supernatural in character, it follows that their causes and cures are beyond the ken of secular healers, who would therefore have been prepared to refrain from hard-nosed inquiry into their nature by genuine (not necessarily priest-imposed) awe of diseases.

Deluged by incessant advertising and propaganda about medical treatments, people forget that Christianity is not only a faith of redemption but also a faith of healing, of both body and soul. Unlike Abraham, Jesus is not only a prophet, he is also a healer, the Divine Physician, the Savior (*der Heiland*, in German). For centuries, Christians regarded sickness as punishment for sin, curable by means of prayer, repentance, sacrifice, and the aspersion of holy water by a priest, the representative of an all-forgiving deity.

To be plague-stricken was to be smitten by God. This put people in a bind: They believed in the theological explanation of the "plague," at least in part, because they could not get at the natural, physical cause of it, and then they refrained from trying to get at the root of the evil because they thought the evil was brought on by the hand of God. Furthermore, everyday life was replete with proof of the efficacy of miraculous cures for illnesses of all kinds. Shrines with powers of healing dotted the Christian landscape. More than 5 million pilgrims a year still visit Lourdes, and, to this day, the Vatican's official procedure for sanctification depends on *medical proof* of the would-be saint's having performed at least two miraculous cures.

We have specific chemicals for specific diseases. Christians had (and still have) specific saints for curing specific ailments. The martyred twins, Cosmas and Damian (c. 303) were the patron saints of medicine in general. St. Vitus had powers to cure chorea (St. Vitus' dance), St. Anthony, to cure erysipelas (Anthony's fire), and St. Rochus, to cure the plague. When Christian monarchs were revered as quasi-divine, their touch was considered curative, especially for scrofula. Revealingly, until c. 1700, the French king would say: *"Le roi te touche, Dieu te guérit"* ("The king touches you, God cures you"). In the eighteenth century, the magic mantra was modified: The king would say: *"Le roi te touche, Dieu te guérisse"* ("The king touches you, may God cure you").

The laying on of hands was transformed into a pseudoscientific "system" by Franz Anton Mesmer (1733–1815): He laid on his hands, and magnetism cured. Before long, the healing power of magnetism was replaced by the healing power of "hypnosis." Mesmer's name has become a part of our language and his work forms both a spiritual and materialist bridge between what I consider magical, ceremonial, or personal healing on the one hand, and material, scientific, and impersonal treatment on the other.[6]

In short, prior to the nineteenth century, neither physicians nor patients had a precise idea about what was and what was not a disease. Disease was simply a discomfort and a danger, often leading to death, to be avoided and relieved as best one could. For centuries, self-medication with herbal remedies—principally opium, alcohol, and tobacco—constituted the suffering person's main protection against illness and pain. As the taboo against treating the body slowly lifted, there arose diverse corps of professional healers: barber surgeons performing operations; herbalists prescribing medicines derived from plants; and doctors of medicine relying mainly on purging the body of presumed toxic substances believed to be the causes of disease.

Among secular healers, barber surgeons were perhaps the most scientific, because their procedures were empirical, and physicians the least scientific, because their procedures were speculative. In fact, the mentality of the prescientific physician was essentially magical-religious, but he applied his craft to the sufferer's vile body, rather than to his wicked soul. This accounts for the jealous rivalry between priest and physician, and the absence of such rivalry between priest and barber surgeon. The persistence of the mystical-religious, Galenic-humoral image of illness right up to the nineteenth century also accounts for the long popularity of premodern medicine's panacea, purging—epitomized by bloodletting. Those who believed in such ideas and interventions worshiped them as rational cure-alls; those who did not, dismissed them as foolish quackeries.

The Core Concept of Disease: The Body as a Machine

The waning influence of religion and the waxing prestige of science were slow and gradual processes. In the sixteenth century, the Church began to authorize the dissection of executed felons. Although physicians participated in this enterprise, the true fathers of anatomy were the great Renaissance artists, especially Michelangelo and Leonardo da Vinci.

The birth of anatomy, as the basis of scientific medicine, is usually attributed to Andreas Witing, a physician from Wesel on the Rhine, better known by his Latin name, Vesalius. In 1543, Vesalius, a professor of anatomy at the University of Padua, published *De humani corporis fabrica* [*The Makeup of the Human Body*]: for the first time in history, people were able to "see, in beautiful and accurate illustrations, the structure of their own bodies."[7] The work made Vesalius famous as well as infamous: He incurred the wrath of the Inquisition and was sentenced to a pilgrimage to the Holy Land, "which, because of the uncertainties of travel at that time, practically amounted to the death penalty; indeed, he never came back from the trip."[8]

Once the secrets of nature are revealed, they cannot be ignored. Physicians and lay persons alike began to view the human body as a machine whose workings must be understood, rather than merely manipulated in the tradition of the herbal empiricists. The stage was now set for the development of the *scientific diagnosis* of patients, both dead and alive. The diagnosis of live patients is a surprisingly recent development. The first diagnostic method, thoracic percussion, was discovered in 1756 by Leopold Auenbrugger (1722–1809), the son of an innkeeper in Graz, Austria. As a youngster, Auenbrugger learned to tap caskets of wine to determine the quantity of liquid in the container and applied the technique to the human chest. This simple but ingenious method led the famed French physician, René-Théophile-Hyacinthe Laennec (1781–1826) to hit on the idea of thoracic auscultation and, in 1816, to the invention of the stethoscope. Although standard thermometric values were developed in the seventeenth century, the systematic measurement of body temperature was introduced into medicine only in 1851.[9] The development of an ever-growing array of diagnostic instruments and techniques followed quickly. Today, the practicing physician can diagnose many diseases in the living patient as objectively and almost as effectively as the pathologist can diagnose them at autopsy. The long-standing gap between antemortem (clinical) diagnosis and postmortem (autopsy) diagnosis has narrowed but has not disappeared. Despite modern diagnostic techniques, the postmortem examination of the cadaver remains an *indispensable* tool for scientific medicine and forensic pathology.

After steady advances in anatomy and physiology, the dawn of the nineteenth century found European and American society confronted with a dilemma. As medical schools multiplied, the demand for corpses as instructional materials for students and surgeons escalated. Because the legal supply of cadavers was unable to meet this demand, a brisk business in black market cadavers arose. "Resurrectionists" dug up recently interred bodies and even manufactured cadavers by "euthanizing" vagrants. In 1831, the Commonwealth of Massachusetts, and in 1832, the British Parliament passed the so-called "Anatomy Acts," which permitted the use of unclaimed bodies for dissection by specially licensed teachers.

Although the development of the modern, scientific concept of disease was a gradual process, the publication, in 1858, of *Cellular Pathology as Based upon Physiological and Pathological Histology,* by Rudolf Virchow (1821–1902), is generally accepted as signaling the birth of modern medicine as a profession based on empirical science. The study of pathology as the phenomenology of disease, combined with the study of bacteriology as the etiology of infectious disease, placed medicine as the *study of bodily disease* on the rock-solid foundation of modern science.

From Gnosis to Diagnosis: *Cui Bono?*

Textbooks of medicine, and especially of pathology, treat diseases as defects and malfunctions of the human body, "bad things" that no "sane" person would wish upon himself. Viewing disease existentially reveals a different landscape. People often assert that they are ill or that another person is sick. It is an error to believe that people say these things only because they have a disease or only because the person they call sick has a disease. People are often sick but do not say so or say so only to a few confidants, and they often assert, for a variety of reasons, that others—about whom they know next to nothing—are sick: thus, people simulate illness or malinger (to avoid military service), simulate health or deny illness (to avoid medical attention), and claim that others are sick by diagnosing them (to justify treating them as patients). These elementary truths have not been lost on artists, who provide us with perceptive accounts of the often complex and devious motives of patients and doctors.[10]

Having a demonstrable disease is not enough to explain why the subject asserts that he is ill (assumes the sick role) or why others assert that he is ill (place him in the sick role). To understand the myriad nonmedical meanings and consequences of illness—that is, the *tactical* rather than descriptive *uses* of terms such as "ill" and "patient"—we must, at least temporarily, ignore the pathological dimensions of the concept and instead focus on the classic problem, *Cui bono?* Cicero explained the importance of posing this question, primarily to oneself, as follows: "When trying a case [the famous judge] L. Cassius never failed to inquire, 'Who gained by it?' Man's character is such that no man undertakes crimes without hope of gain." ("*L. Cassius . . . in causis quaerere solebat 'cui bono' fuisset. Sic vita hominum est, ut ad maleficium nemo conetur sine spe atque emolumento accedere."* Marcus Tullius Cicero, 106–43 B.C.)[11]

No man asserts that he or someone else has an illness without hope of gain. The potential gains, for oneself or others, from asserting such a claim—for example, securing medical help, monetary compensation, excusing crime, and so forth—are virtually endless. They depend on the claimant's character and motives, the social context in which the claim is advanced, and the ever-changing legal and social milieu in which medicine is practiced.

In this book, I shall use the terms "disease," "discomfort," and "deviance" in specific and distinct ways. Disease refers to a demonstrable alteration in the structure or function of the body as a material object considered harmful to the organism, for example, a cancerous lesion or paralysis as a result of a stroke. Discomfort denotes the complaint of an individual about his own body and behavior, for example, pain, fatigue, or depression. Finally, deviance identifies the complaint of individuals about the behaviors of other persons or groups, for example, the habitual use of legal or illegal drugs, illegal sexual behavior, or behavior causing injury or death to others or the self.

If we count discomforts and deviances as diseases, we change the criterion for what counts as a disease and set the ground for steadily expanding the category called "disease." Patients suffering from discomforts can classify their feelings of malaise as diseases and can try to convince others to accept their claims. Many prominent persons now engage in this kind of disease promotion: some advertise their depression as a brain disease, others their impotence as ED (erectile dysfunction), still others their former drug use from which they are "in recovery." Physicians and politicians can do the same with other people's deviance. Because physicians and politicians regularly function as agents of the therapeutic state, this is an ominous development: acting in concert, they possess the power needed to convince, coerce, co-opt, or corrupt the public to accept the *illness inflation* they promote.

This process of illness inflation—or, more precisely, diagnosis inflation—began in the seventeenth century with the postmortem diagnosis of suicides as *non compos mentis*, hence excusable for their felonious deed of self-murder.[12] It gathered speed in the eighteenth and nineteenth centuries with the medicalization of crime and sex, exemplified by the popularization of the insanity defense, the hospitalization of the insane, and the fabrication of diagnoses such as masturbatory insanity.[13] And it is now running amok, virtually every wrenching personal experience and socially undesirable behavior being diagnosed as a disease and discovered to be treatable by an intervention classified as health care.

2

SCIENTIFIC MEDICINE
Disease

Scientific medicine has as its object the discovery of changed conditions characterizing the sick body or the individual suffering organ.

Rudolf Virchow (1821–1902)[1]

The necropsy is, and remains, the final, crucial, common pathway in "disease." . . . [It] is of fundamental importance and irreplaceable in medical science.

Alvan R. Feinstein (1967)[2]

When patients die, autopsy is considered to be the optimal standard to confirm clinical diagnoses.

John Roosen et al. (2000)[3]

Before there was science, there was religion, and before there was scientific medicine, there was magical medicine. For a long time, people attributed medical powers to priests, the priests believed they possessed such powers, and the temporal rulers legitimized priests as effective healers. Today, people tend to attribute near-magical powers to physicians, many physicians believe they possess such powers, and the state legitimizes physicians as effective healers. What counts or ought to count as a disease (or treatment) forms no part of these systems of belief.

Magical medicine men—from primitive shamans with painted faces to modern charlatans puffed on television—can cure diseases they can neither clearly define nor objectively identify. Scientific medicine men—exemplified by the pioneer pathologists who sought to define and objectively identify *disease*, before trying to explain *it*, let alone trying to remedy *it*—promise no such miracles. We must not lose sight of this ironic disjunction between knowing what a disease is, and knowing how to relieve the patient of suffering; if we forget it, we are likely to yield to the temptation to think of disease in terms of it being "treatable," by an officially accredited expert, by an officially accredited method.

John Selden, a seventeenth-century English jurist and scholar, warned: "The reason of a thing is not to be inquired after, till you are sure the thing itself be so. We commonly are at, *what's the reason for it?* before we are sure of the thing."[4] If we fail to heed this principle, we risk "explaining" a troubling phenomenon—for example, the plague or schizophrenia—without knowing precisely what the thing is that we are explaining.

THE CONCEPT OF DISEASE

The concept of disease as an affliction of living organisms is probably as old as civilization. With the dawn of human consciousness, people must have noticed that plants, animals, and human beings sometimes change their appearance, lose their normal functions, wither, and die. They also must have noticed that this process often affects many of the same organisms at the same time or in rapid succession. Consider the following scriptural account of an epidemic created deliberately by a kind of bacterial warfare: "And the Lord said unto Moses and unto Aaron, Take to you handfuls of ashes of the furnace, and let Moses sprinkle it toward the heaven in the sight of Pharaoh. And it shall become small dust in all the land of Egypt, and shall be a boil breaking forth with blains upon man, and upon beast, throughout all the land of Egypt."[5]

Whether this epidemic, affecting both man and beast, was anthrax is speculation, but it may well have been. Anthrax is one of the oldest known diseases of animals; its manifestations were recorded by Homer, Hippocrates, Galen, and Pliny.[6] The microbe *Bacillus anthracis* can infect dogs, cats, cattle, sheep, goats, horses, mules, and swine. It is the first infectious disease against which a vaccine was developed, by Louis Pasteur in 1881.

Ever since antiquity, historians have recorded plagues destroying armies and cities; leprosy and venereal diseases have long been understood to be "contagious," that is, spread by human contact.[7] People grasped the idea of contagion long before the discovery of microscopic organisms. What people did not grasp, even long after their discovery, was that these organisms could harm human beings.

People abhor being baffled by the dangers that face them. Preferring a false explanation to none, most people want, and are relatively easily satisfied with, any "plausible" explanation for everything they fear. Thus, people knew, or thought they knew, that the plague was caused by demons, witches, the breaking of taboo, the evil eye, humoral imbalance, Jews poisoning wells, and so forth, and that it could be cured by exorcism, aspersion of holy water, bloodletting, worthless herbal medicine, and so forth. One reason for the late development of the scientific concept of disease was, as I noted earlier, the ready availability of false explanations; another was the lag in the application of science to medicine.[8]

The Core Concept of Disease: Somatic Pathology

Religion tells us that the mortal human body is a vessel, given to us by God, to house our immortal soul. Science tells us that the body is a biological machine that we inhabit and use, but whose structure and function we do not fully understand. This perspective—which makes it plausible to compare understanding the makeup of the body as a machine and fixing its breakdowns to understanding the makeup of a complex man-made machine and fixing its breakdowns—has profound implications for the concept of disease and for medicine as science and technology.

We know how to use cars, computers, television sets, and many other machines, without necessarily understanding their internal structures and functions, let alone knowing how to fix them when they break down. However, there are experts who know how to make and repair such machines. Those experts need precise definitions for certain terms for practicing their craft competently, and it is they who typically define the meaning of terms that refer to objects or practices used in their daily work. For example, the word "muffler" means one thing to an auto mechanic and another thing to a haberdasher. The same goes for the word "disease." For pathologists, disease is a bodily lesion, something they can observe, objectively demonstrate, perhaps even deliberately reproduce. For practicing physicians, it is the malady from which they think the patient suffers. For patients, disease is the condition to which they attribute feeling unwell. For psychiatrists, politicians, journalists, and people generally, it is all of the above and anything else they want to make it.

Each of these concepts has its proper place. But only the pathologist's concept of disease is *relevant* to the scientific definition of disease as a *departure from normal bodily structure and function.* "All illnesses," writes Stanley L. Robbins, the author of a standard textbook of pathology, "are expressions of cellular derangements."[9] This concept is indifferent to the condition's cause, the affected organism's feelings or wishes about it, or society's legal and political attitude toward it. For example, a malignancy, say cancer of the lung, is not a disease because the patient coughs up blood (a sign of disease); and an injury, say whiplash as a result of a traffic accident, is not a disease because it results in disability and is a source of monetary compensation (consequences of disease). René Leriche (1874–1955), famous French surgeon and founder of modern vascular surgery, was right when he observed, with something of a rhetorical flourish: "If one wants to define disease it must be dehumanized. . . . In disease, when all is said and done, the least important thing is man."[10]

In this connection, it cannot be overemphasized that while a particular pattern of behavior may be the cause or the consequence of a disease, *the behavior, per se, cannot, as a matter of definition, be a disease.* Boxing or drinking alcohol may cause diseases but are not diseases. Disability—the inability to earn a living or care for oneself—may be, or may not be, a consequence of disease, but is not a disease.

The importance of a purely materialist-scientific definition of disease is perhaps best appreciated by comparing it to the purely materialist-scientific definition of, say, carbon. The carbon atom has certain specific physical properties that distinguish it from every other element. Those properties are physical, not economic or technological. Coal and diamond are two kinds of carbon, much as diabetes and diphtheria are two kinds of disease. To the untrained eye and uninformed mind, these phenomena are grossly dissimilar. Yet, to the trained eye and informed mind, they are members of the same class: carbon and disease, respectively.

The economic value or social uses of coal and diamond are not relevant to the concept of carbon, as a term of scientific discourse. We do not infer what a substance is from its value or use. Gold, like diamond, is valuable and used as jewelry, but we do not infer from this that it *is composed of carbon.*

Similarly, the therapeutic implications of diabetes and diphtheria are not relevant to the *concept* of disease, as a term of scientific discourse. We do not, as a rule, infer what a disease is from its response to treatment. Like diabetes, depression—psychiatrists say—is "treatable." That does not entitle them to claim that depression is a disease. (Diabetes was, of course, a disease before it was treatable.)

RUDOLF VIRCHOW: IDENTIFYING DISEASE

Medical historians view Virchow (1821–1902) as the Newton (1642–1727) of scientific medicine. Emanuel Rubin and John L. Farber, the authors of the textbook *Pathology,* state: "Rudolf Virchow, often referred to as the father of modern pathology . . . propos(ed) that the basis of all disease is injury to the smallest living unit of the body, namely, the cell. More than a century later, both clinical and experimental pathology remain rooted in Virchow's cellular pathology."[11] Alvan R. Feinstein, professor of medicine at Yale medical school, declares: "Virchow's work was magnificent, laying the foundation on which modern histopathology still rests, and demolishing the erroneous doctrine of humoral causes for disease."[12] David M. Reese, an oncologist at the University of California at Los Angeles, writes: "Like Newton's *Principia* two centuries earlier, the work [Virchow's *Die Cellular- pathologie*] caused an immediate sensation in Europe. Theories about disease now could be unified under a single rubric, the concept of the cell and its normal and pathological functioning."[13]

The identification of disease as a physical-chemical phenomenon is contingent—as is the identification of any other such phenomenon—on the method of observation available to the investigator. For the pioneer anatomical pathologists, disease was an abnormal organ visible to the naked eye. The microscope and tissue-staining techniques enabled physicians to examine tissues and cells and led to the distinction between anatomy and histology, gross pathology and microscopic pathology (histopathology). With the development of each new technology—from the x-ray and electrocardiograph to chemical and serological tests—the *methods* used to detect disease were widened: The detection-identification of disease may thus be morphological, histological, radiological, chemical, serological, and so forth. However, the criterion of disease remains the same: functional or structural abnormality of cells, tissues, or organs. In this book, I repeatedly contrast bodily diseases with so-called mental diseases, which I classify as nondiseases. Because the mind is not a bodily organ, it can be diseased only in a metaphorical sense. Since there is no objective method for detecting the presence of mental illness, there is also no such method for establishing its absence. The claim that a mental illness is a brain disease is profoundly self-contradictory: a disease of the brain is a brain disease, not a mental disease.

Medical scientists are, of course, not satisfied with identifying diseases; they want to identify their causes as well. Besides chemical and physical injuries, the most obvious causes of disease are infections. As a result, the scientific identification of disease has always been partly descriptive and partly explanatory. The diagnosis "squamous cell carcinoma" is an example of a descriptive diagnostic term, requiring microscopic examination of the tissue for definitive identification, whereas the diagnosis "vitamin C deficiency"—which replaced the term "scurvy," a descriptive diagnosis—is an etiological diagnostic term.

Disease as Cellular Pathology

The definition of disease as cellular pathology is an idea that, as medical historian Erwin H. Ackerknecht put it, "has dominated biology and pathology up to this very day."[14] Why was this idea so fundamental to the development of medicine as a science? Because prior to the cellular-pathological concept of disease, there were many theories of disease, so-called "systems." However, none was based on empirically verifiable observations or served the interest of advancing knowledge; instead, each served the interests of its promoter, creating famed healers and founders of systems, such as Galen and Paracelsus, Mesmer and Freud. This model of disease theorizing continued after Virchow in the field of psychiatry, exemplified by the system created by Emil Kraepelin and its progeny, the periodically revised versions of the American Psychiatric Association's *Diagnostic and Statistical Manual of Mental Disorders* (*DSM*s).

Born in a small town in Prussia, trained as a physician, Virchow's first job was dissecting corpses at the morgue of the *Charité*, the prestigious, municipal teaching hospital in Berlin. His concept of disease was firmly anchored in the context of that experience. Disease was not what the patient complained of, nor was it what the physician at the bedside observed. Disease was not defined in terms of its cause or cure. Instead, it was identified in terms of what the pathologist could detect in cells, tissues, and organs, at autopsy or, in the case of the living person, in a biopsy specimen surgically removed from his body.

Virchow's concept of disease was thus *phenomenological*, in the scientific, not the philosophical, sense of that word. In 1845, when Virchow was only twenty-four years old and barely two years after receiving his medical degree, he formulated the idea that was to become the core concept of disease. In an address titled "On the Need and Correctness of a Medicine Based on a Mechanistic Approach," he argued that "the goal of modern medicine should be to establish firmly *a physics of organisms according to mechanical laws, with the cell as the organic molecule, analogous to the chemical or physical atom.*"[15] By observing an apple falling to the ground, Newton identified and defined gravity. By observing "abnormal" cells, tissues, and organs, Virchow identified and defined disease. The apple has no opinion about gravity. The cadaver or the patient's body has no voice about disease. We have forgotten this simple fact and are paying dearly for our amnesia.

When we treat medicine as a science, similar to the hard sciences, the implications are far reaching. Just as physical science deprived the popes of their authority regarding the movement of planets, so medical science deprives patients—as well as priests and politicians—of their authority regarding the definition, nature, cause, and cure of disease. This development is not something to regret, but something to celebrate. Authority over the scientific definition of disease must not be confused with authority for judging the ethics of medical interventions or the power to provide or prohibit such interventions.

As noted at the head of this chapter, in Virchow's view the object of scientific medicine is "the discovery of changed conditions, characterizing the sick *body* or the individual suffering *organ*." To this he added that "its foundation is thus physiology."[16] As a science, medicine qua pathology is thus *materialistic*. Virchow put it thus: "This science [pathology], which naturally includes a cellular theory of the living, proceeds from the fact that cells are the actual operative parts of the body.... The same substance [cells], which is the bearer of life, is also the bearer of sickness. *Every spiritualistic impulse is excluded*."[17]

Virchow anticipated the confusion, common today, between disease per se and the etiology of disease as contributory cause (along with the host organism's reaction to it), but not disease per se: "It thus happens, as I have repeatedly set forth, that there is the confusion of a being with a cause, of an *ens morbi* with a *causa morbi*. An actual parasite ... can be the cause of a disease, but it can never exhibit the disease itself."[18] Cancer of the lung is a disease. But smoking—even if diagnosed as "nicotine dependence" or "substance abuse"—is not and cannot be a disease, just as a microorganism per se is not and cannot be a disease.

Virchow never deviated from the concept of disease as phenomenon, independent of its etiology or explanation. "The secret of disease," concluded medical popularizer Rene Dubos, "appeared to reside in the anatomy of the tissues."[19] It was not only the secret of disease that resided there, its definition did as well.

Virchow as Social Activist

The publication of Virchow's *Cellular Pathology* in 1858 established "his reputation as the founder of a new scientific discipline."[20] What scientific discipline? *Medicine as a science.* However, medicine was then, and is now, a personal service as well as a scientific activity. The service component—which we call "clinical medicine" or "medical practice" and which often overshadows the scientific foundation of medicine—is not, and cannot be, a science. Why? Because its goal is to increase the well-being of the patient, whereas the goal of scientific medicine is to increase our knowledge about the nature of the human body in health and disease. The well-being of the patient is not a fact, but an opinion or judgment, not necessarily the patient's; it may be the opinion of a parent or guardian, a judge, or a health maintenance organization (HMO). Thus, while the valuation of disease as something undesirable is central to the clinical concept of disease, it is only peripheral to its scientific concept. (The prefix "dis" is not merely descriptive but also, *eo ipso*, negatively valuative.)

Although Virchow was a superb observer, by temperament he was not a reclusive scientist, satisfied with exploring a limited aspect of the world from within the sanctuary of his laboratory. Recognizing what was obvious then and is obvious now, namely, that poor people are more likely to be afflicted with diseases than rich people, Virchow became a medical and social revolutionary in the fashion of the French *philosophes*.[21] He fought against the alliance of the church and the state and wanted to replace it by an alliance of science, especially medicine, and the state. The abolition of poverty by politics and of ignorance by education promised a utopian future. Indeed, it was Virchow who, in 1873, coined the term *Kulturkampf*—literally, struggle for culture, here used to refer to the conflict between the secular-scientific and religious-mystical world views and, more specifically, to the political struggle against the influence of the Catholic church in Prussian politics: "He sincerely believed that the church . . . was incompatible with modern natural science and indeed with fundamental principles of freedom, tolerance, and rationality that had been the foundations of secular society in Western Europe since the Enlightenment. . . . He boldly stated that in the modern age science rather than religion would provide the basis for morality."[22]

A political naif, Virchow had not the slightest understanding of the dependence of individual liberty on the security of property, the rule of law, and the checks that, in a secular society, the church and other informal organizations provide against unlimited state power. Thus, not only was Virchow the founder of the scientific concept of disease, he was also an early and enthusiastic supporter of the therapeutic state. Unaware that treating certain aspects of the human condition as if they were diseases is full of pitfalls, he agitated for "school hygiene" and declared that "the whole penitentiary system was . . . actually a public health problem. Punishment should be replaced with psychiatric education."[23]

In 1871, after the defeat of the French in the Franco-Prussian war, Virchow claimed that the war had been "forced on Prussia" and quoted approvingly the opinion of the German psychiatrist Karl Stark, "that at the time the war broke out the French might have been gripped by some form of collective insanity."[24] These remarks foreshadow the denunciation—couched in a diagnostic vocabulary—of Jews as genetic degenerates, of Hitler and other despots as psychopaths, and similar semantic assaults masquerading as medical diagnoses. Evidently, it never occurred to Virchow that medical statism could be just as inimical to individual liberty as religious statism.

With respect to mixing science and theology, Virchow's scientific convictions served him well. In 1868, a Belgian novitiate was supposed to have miraculously survived for three years with "no sustenance except water and the communion host." Asked by the Vatican to examine the woman and render an expert medical opinion about the claim, Virchow recognized that there was nothing to examine and refused.[25] However, his scientific convictions failed him with respect to mixing science and politics: his compassion for the poor led him to flirt with medical statism, and his desire to please authority contributed to his worst blunder as a scientist.

Shortly before becoming emperor for the last ninety-nine days of his life, Crown Prince Frederick III (1831–1888) complained of hoarseness. His physician found a small growth on one of his vocal cords and treated it with electrocoagulation. Soon the growth recurred and malignancy was suspected. Surgical excision of the tumor, requiring removal of the larynx, was considered life-threatening and, even if successful, would have resulted in the loss of his voice, incapacitating him for the role of emperor. To resolve the dilemma and since the crown princess was English, the most prominent English throat specialist, Dr. Morell Mackenzie, was called for consultation. Dr. Mackenzie decided that a correct diagnosis required examining a biopsy specimen of the affected tissue. Naturally, the task of examining the tissue and rendering a final diagnosis fell upon the shoulders of Rudolf Virchow, the most famous pathologist in the world. Mindful of political power, Virchow, it appears, did not want to be the bearer of a fatal prognosis: "He declared that all of the growth was located on the surface . . . unlike malignancies. . . . Labeling the illness *Pachydermia laryngis vericosa* [a wart on the larynx], he said that the generally healthy condition of the tissue gave a very good prognosis."[26] As a result, Mackenzie had no reason to remove the tumor. The lesion was malignant. Three months later Frederick was dead. The autopsy, conducted by Virchow in the presence of Mackenzie and the emperor's personal physicians, revealed that "the larynx was completely destroyed through cancer and putrid bronchitis."[27] Recriminations among the physicians who had attended the emperor now ensued, Virchow being accused of failing to examine the patient, confining himself to examining only the biopsy specimen. Virchow in turn accused Mackenzie of having taken the biopsy from the healthy part of the larynx. In the end, Virchow escaped with his reputation unblemished.

LOUIS PASTEUR: EXPLAINING DISEASE

Understanding Pasteur's contribution to medicine as a science requires that we recapture the pre-Darwinian scientific view regarding the nature of living matter. Before biology could become a science, biologists had to answer the question, What is the origin of life? The biblical answer was that God created all things, nonliving and living, including man. The scientific answer, in Pasteur's day, was called "spontaneous generation"; that is, under certain conditions not yet understood, living organisms arose "spontaneously" from nonliving matter: "Under a thousand symbols, men of all religions and philosophies have sung and portrayed the repeated emergence of life from inanimate matter."[28] This idea, now as discredited as the idea that the earth is flat, was ardently supported by Pasteur's contemporaries.

Disease and the Struggle for Life

Since earliest times, people must have recognized that many animals live off other animals. Wrote Jonathan Swift (1667–1745): "So, naturalists observe, a flea / Has smaller fleas that on him prey; / And these have smaller still to bite 'em; / And so proceed *ad infinitum*."[29] Anthropologists believe that the initial impetus for civilization through cooperation may have been man's desire to avoid becoming food.

People must have also recognized that once living beings die, their remains "turn to dust," as the Bible phrased it. How does that happen? It happens by dead bodies becoming food for animals that require "living matter" for sustenance, for example, vultures feeding off carrion. It remained for Pasteur to demonstrate that this process—animals "eating" other animals—occurs on a microscopic level as well. He thus brought home to mankind—and especially to medical scientists—that human beings are consumed not only by animals we can see with the naked eye but also by "animals" we cannot see without the aid of the microscope. This laid the ground for formulating the fundamental *etiological* core of the concept of disease—namely, the destruction of the body of a living host (plant or animal) by pathogenic microorganisms. In hindsight, this discovery came astonishingly late in the history of science.

Using a microscope, the great Dutch naturalist Anton Leeuwenhoek (1632–1723) had demonstrated the existence of microorganisms—"little animals"—seemingly everywhere in nature. However, for nearly 200 years, this discovery made no impact on physicians. The anatomist pioneers of modern medicine were interested in identifying *lesions* that correlated with clinical diseases; they were not concerned with the etiology or pathogenesis of disease. This underscores how far we have moved in the opposite direction: today, leaders in medicine are far more interested in *naming a cause*—for every aspect of the human condition—than in finding a new lesion. The understanding of disease as a biological—chemical and microbial—process had to wait until 1857, when Pasteur published his seemingly unrelated classic studies on fermentation.

To grasp the nature of light as both corpuscular and wave-like, physicists had to reject the existence of the ether—that is, the notion that space is filled with minute invisible particles of matter. Similarly, to grasp that life can arise only from living matter, biologists had to reject the existence of spontaneous generation—that is, the notion that life can arise, de novo, from nonliving matter. By the same token, to grasp the nature of human conflict and its potentially horrifying consequences, we must reject the notion that (unwanted) behavior can be a real disease.

Pasteur was not a physician. He had no medical training whatever. Pasteur was a chemist who spent the first ten years of his scientific career, from 1847 to 1857, laying the groundwork for the field known as stereochemistry. He became one of the founding fathers of scientific medicine by a lucky accident—being asked to solve the problem of silkworm disease. Luck, however, as he later remarked, "favors the prepared mind."

Along with cotton and wool, silk had long been one of the most useful fibers known to man. The material comes from the secretion of the mulberry leaf-feeding silkworm, *Bombyx mori*, a family of Lepidoptera that includes large moths and butterflies. The mature caterpillar produces a clear, viscous fluid called fibroin, which, in combination with another fluid called sericin, forms the solid filaments of silk that make up the cocoon.

Silk has been used since antiquity. Long before Pasteur's time, many countries, including France, had flourishing silkworm industries. People who made a living cultivating silkworms were familiar with the fact that silkworms sometimes failed to develop proper cocoons and hence yielded little or no usable fibers. No one knew what caused the problem, called "disease of silkworms" (*pébrine*, in French), nor did anyone have a remedy for it. The only thing the grower affected by this problem could do was to destroy the affected worms and start all over with batches of healthy worms. As is usually the case with authorities who have no understanding of a problem, the experts had many explanations for silkworm disease, ranging from poor-quality mulberry leaves to improper humidity and temperature levels in the silkworm incubators.

Actually, an amateur scientist in Italy, Agostino Bassi (1773–1856), had discovered the cause and nature of silkworm disease more than twenty years before Pasteur rediscovered it. In 1853, Bassi published his classic monograph, *Del Mal del Segno*[30] (the Italian name for silkworm disease), showing that the ailment was infectious, caused by a microscopic parasitic fungus transmitted from one silkworm to another by direct contact or through infected food.

Bassi was trained as a lawyer but, like many great nineteenth-century scientists, his health was said to be too poor to permit him to practice his profession. However, he lived to be eighty-three and spent his life as a gentleman scholar. Although he lacked training or even interest in medicine or veterinary science, he—more than Pasteur or Koch—is the true father of the germ theory of disease. Because Bassi was an amateur, during his lifetime his discovery was ignored by experts on silkworm disease as well as by medical scientists. After his death, his work was overshadowed by that of Pasteur, Robert Koch, and the other pioneers of bacteriology. The *Encyclopaedia Britannica* devotes only two brief paragraphs to Bassi's life and his work. However, the organism he discovered is named *Botrytis bassiana*.

By the middle of the nineteenth century, the French silkworm industry was virtually in ruins. Silkworm disease spread to Italy, Spain, and Austria, and eventually to China and Japan. In 1865, Jean Baptiste André Dumas (1800–1884)—one of the world's preeminent chemists—requested and received authorization from the Minister of Agriculture to appoint a mission to study *pébrine*.[31] Dumas, who had been Pasteur's teacher and scientific mentor, asked his pupil to investigate the problem. Until that day, Pasteur had never seen a silkworm or a mulberry tree, the leaves of which served as food for the worms. As legend has it, Pasteur—who knew nothing about the subject and evidently wanted to demur—inquired: "Is there then a disease of silkworms?" To which, Dumas replied: "So much the better! For ideas you will have only those which shall come to you as a result of your own observations!"[32]

When Pasteur undertook to investigate the disease, he had already made a monumental discovery that proved extremely useful. It had long been known that when organic matter is left alone, it undergoes a seemingly spontaneous transformation. Why and how this happened, however, was not known. Understanding the process was hampered by its having two different names: if it involved the conversion of sugars and starches into alcohols, it was called "fermentation," but if it involved the decomposition of proteins into foul-smelling products, it was called "putrefaction." We still use these terms. But, thanks to Pasteur, we now understand that the production of beer and the production of pus rest on similar principles and processes.

Knowing that something occurs or making use of that knowledge is a far cry from *understanding* how and why it happens. That was the case with fermentation and putrefaction until Pasteur came along. Since antiquity, people knew how to make bread from starch, and wine from grape juice. Because these processes are accompanied by the formation of carbon dioxide gas causing bubbling in the product, bread and wine became the symbols of life.

People also knew that organic matter decomposed, dead bodies turning to dust. It was to combat this process that ancient Egyptians developed the art of embalming. However, it is unlikely that they realized that if dead plants and animals did not decompose—becoming a part of the soil, the air, and the water—their remains would soon cover the surface of the earth. It remained for Pasteur to discover that fermentation and putrefaction are similar chemical processes, each depending on a catalyst, yeast, that is necessary for, but is not an active participant in, the reactions.

After studying the problem for six years, in 1861 Pasteur reported that fermentation and putrefaction were both caused by living organisms. This discovery spelled the doom of the theory of spontaneous generation, a sacrosanct doctrine that had hobbled the development of biology for centuries. In the course of arriving at this conclusion, Pasteur made another basic discovery: He showed that many biochemical processes are anaerobic; that is, they can occur only in the absence of air (oxygen). He observed that although the yeast organism necessary for fermentation grows most rapidly in the presence of air, it produces fermentation most efficiently in its absence. These discoveries gained Pasteur the recognition he so richly deserved. The term "pasteurization"—identifying the process of preventing unwanted fermentation ("spoilage") by controlled heating—has become a verb in virtually all modern languages.

What, exactly, is the relevance of fermentation to disease? Dubos answered the question as follows:

> The concepts dealing with fermentation and contagious diseases followed a parallel evolution during the two centuries which followed Boyle's statement. In both cases, two opposite doctrines competed for the explanation of observed phenomena. According to one, the primary motive force—be it of fermentation, putrefaction, or disease—resided in the altered body itself, being either self-generated or induced by some *chemical* force which set the process in motion. According to the other doctrine, the process was caused by an independent, *living agent*, foreign in nature and origin to the body undergoing the alteration, and *living in it as a parasite*. It is the conflict between these doctrines which gives an internal unity to the story of Pasteur's scientific life.[33]

Thus, when Pasteur undertook to investigate silkworm disease, he was mentally prepared to assume that it might be caused by a microorganism, which is precisely what he found. By examining the silkworm eggs under a microscope, infected eggs could be easily separated from uninfected eggs, preventing the production of additional diseased worms and the perpetuation of the disease.

Pasteur's discovery of the nature of silkworm disease had a powerful impact on shaping the scientific concept of disease. The idea that disease is a *loss of natural function* antedates modern medicine. Pasteur demonstrated that certain abnormalities of the organism's body, identifiable with the aid of the microscope, may be consistently associated with, and be the markers of, disease. The eggs of diseased silkworms could be easily distinguished from the eggs of healthy silkworms. This understanding was of no help for *curing* the malady, but it enabled breeders to *prevent* the disease by identifying and discarding infected eggs and selecting only healthy eggs for breeding.

It bears emphasizing that, in Pasteur's hands, the identification of diseased silkworm eggs began and ended as an ordinary, commonsense process, rather than as a specialized scientific procedure. To be sure, understanding the disease as a microbial infection was a scientific discovery. However, once that was accomplished, Pasteur made both the diagnosis and the prevention of the disease a commonsense procedure whose mastery required only a simple skill, easily learned by anyone who wished.

DISEASE AS FACT, DISEASE AS JUDGMENT

Once it was recognized that microorganisms could cause disease in silkworms, it was easy to conclude that they might also cause disease in human beings. "The very use of the word 'diseases' (*maladies*) to describe these alterations," Dubos observed, "rendered more obvious the suggestion that microorganisms might also invade human and animal tissues, as they had already been proved to do in the case of silkworms."[34]

The process of animal A feeding on animal B is simply a fact we observe. The element of *value* enters the picture if we intervene or wish to intervene. For example, we can help B by protecting him from being eaten by A: in effect, this is what we do when we take an antibiotic. Penicillin is therapeutic for the patient (whom we want to save), but is toxic for the microorganisms (that we want to destroy). Or, we can help A by providing it with an ample supply of B: this is what we do when we breed animals to feed people. Raising chickens in vast factories is good for us: it provides us with a source of abundant, nutritious food. But the enterprise is bad for chickens: it creates huge numbers of them, raised in cramped quarters, for the sole purpose of being eaten.

The image of illness as a combat, with the victorious animal eating his victim, dramatizes the element of *valuation* intrinsic to the concept of disease. It was this image that impressed itself on Pasteur's mind, guided all of his medical work, and inspired him to suggest that "septicemia may be termed a putrefaction of the living organism."[35]

Actually, the evaluative element in the concept of disease is self-evident. Pasteur was commissioned to work on silkworm disease for a practical reason—to help the silkworm industry to be profitable. The motive for this pioneering piece of medical research was commercial, not compassion for human suffering or disinterested scientific curiosity, let alone the desire to cure sick silkworms.

The understanding of the mechanism of human diseases thus began with the search for controlling certain biological processes that resulted in the destruction of *property*, specifically, animals and plants useful to man—such as anthrax affecting cattle and sheep and phylloxera affecting vine-producing grapes. In the case of anthrax, the phenomenon we deem to be a disease is a struggle between anthrax bacilli and their host, with the microbes winning. Although that account of anthrax is both explanatory and valuative, it is not value-dependent in the sense that we call anthrax in cattle a disease *solely* because we value filet mignon more highly than anthrax bacilli.

From a scientific point of view, we could equally well speak of a disease affecting anthrax bacilli.

In the case of endogenous diseases—say, diabetes or lupus—the valuation lies in the assumption, explicit or tacit, that it is better for a person to live with a normally functioning biological makeup than with a makeup that malfunctions, causing disability and death.[36] "Health," observes medical ethicist Leon Kass, "is a natural standard or norm—not a moral norm, not a 'value' as opposed to a 'fact.' . . . [It is] a state of being that reveals itself in activity as the standard of bodily excellence or fitness relative to each species."[37] Kass correctly emphasizes that the concept of health piggybacks on the concept of disease, which in turn must be located in the body. Disease reveals itself in the *abnormal activity of the body, not of the person.*

That the concept of disease contains an element of value judgment does not diminish the primarily and essentially *descriptive, phenomenological* character of the pathological concept of disease. An element of valuation may be present in certain physical concepts as well. For example, ounce for ounce, helium is more valuable than iron. This does not affect the phenomenological identifications of helium and iron in terms of the number of protons and electrons in their respective atoms. Virchow's achievement is similar. It is important that we distinguish the negative value attached to a particular disease from the concept of disease as a phenomenon. If we fail to do so, we are likely to mistake negative value for disease and classify as diseases phenomena—unwanted behaviors—*that display no evidence of abnormal bodily structure or function.* This is not a supposition or a warning about a hypothetical danger. It is a description of the present medical-social scene: We are in the midst of galloping disease inflation, characterized by an elevation of social judgment to a criterion for diagnosis.

Throughout this book, I maintain that the scientific concept of disease rests on objective standards, in principle similar to those of the physical sciences. In this chapter I rely heavily on Virchow's epochal contributions, especially anchoring the scientific concept of disease in the autopsy, that is, the pathologist's postmortem examination. Some readers may be tempted to find fault with this reasoning, minimizing or even dismissing Virchow's work as outdated or even anachronistic. However, just as Newton's ideas on the concept of gravity remain valid and important, so do Virchow's ideas on the concept of disease.

In June 2000, the *Mayo Clinic Proceedings* published a major study and an editorial reminding us of and reiterating the pivotal role of the autopsy in scientific medicine. The authors, a group of Belgian physicians, compared the clinical diagnoses of 100 randomly selected patients who died in a medical intensive care unit with their autopsy diagnoses, and found that "in 16%, autopsy findings revealed a major diagnosis that, if known before death, might have led to a change in therapy and prolonged survival." They concluded: "Despite the progress of imaging techniques, new tumors are frequently diagnosed at autopsy. . . . Despite the introduction of modern diagnostic techniques and of intensive and invasive monitoring, the number of missed major diagnoses has not essentially changed over the past 20 to 30 years. . . . Our study reaffirms the validity and usefulness of autopsy."[38]

In an accompanying editorial, entitled "The Persistent Importance of Autopsies," G. William Moore and Grover M. Hutchins, pathologists at the University of Maryland and Johns Hopkins University Medical Schools, list the main reasons why the rate of autopsies and reliance on them for final diagnoses have been steadily declining in American hospitals, and reemphasize that postmortem examination remains the basis of scientific medicine. Autopsies are on the decline because of "a false belief that everything important is known about the patient before death; an equally false belief that autopsy findings contribute no understanding of pathophysiologic events in the patient; . . . an increasingly cumbersome physical process of performing autopsies . . . due to increased risk of infectious diseases. . . ." Additionally, physicians sometimes avoid seeking permission for autopsies, lest they show that the clinical diagnosis was mistaken and be used as evidence to support malpractice litigation against them and the hospital: "Not only is this public exposure self-defeating in terms of securing the cooperation of our clinical colleagues in obtaining autopsy permissions, but it does not generally serve to advance the practice of medicine."[39]

CONCLUSIONS

Scientific concepts are defined by scientists and then used, or not used, by people as they deem fit. The fact that the patient plays no role in the scientific definition of disease does not, as some people erroneously believe, diminish his dignity or deprive him of any rights. Authority over the scientific definition of disease must not be confused with power over controlling medical interventions available to people or with authority to judge the ethics of medical research, prevention, or treatment. In a free society, people have a right to think anything they want, including believing that they have a disease even when they don't. Although masculinity and femininity are biological concepts, people are often permitted to define whether they are men or women.[40]

A congenital problem about gender identity occurs in approximately one in 30,000 apparently male births, and in approximately one in 100,000 apparently female births. Most of these people "genuinely believe that they have been ascribed the wrong sex."[41] We recognize that, in such cases, the individuals' gender preferences do not match their chromosomal and/or physical sexual identity. The point is that scientists define gender as independent of the person's physical appearance, sexual self-identification, or sexual identification by other lay persons. *The only scientifically relevant criterion for gender is genetic—that is, chromosomal makeup.*

Similarly, scientists define disease as independent of the person's self-identification as a patient or his identification as a patient by others. *The only scientifically relevant criterion for disease is medical—that is, cellular pathology.* Who says so? Pathologists. The latest edition of *Robbins Pathologic Basis of Disease* (6th edition, 1999)—an authoritative, multiauthor text—defines disease indirectly, by defining the nature and scope of pathology, as follows: "The four aspects of the disease process that form the core of pathology are its cause (etiology), the mechanism of development (pathogenesis), the structural alterations induced in cells and organs (morphologic changes), and the functional consequences of the morphologic changes (clinical significance)."[42]

Accordingly, asserting that a particular person's problem is a disease because the patient or others *believe* it is a disease, or because it *looks* like a disease, or because doctors *diagnose* it as a disease, and treat it with drugs as if it *were* a disease, or because it *entitles the subject to be qualified as disabled,* or because it *presents an economic burden to the subject's family or society*—all that is irrelevant for the scientific concept of disease. Nevertheless, as we shall see time and again, the piling up of such nonsequiturs forms the basis for much of the contemporary confusion and controversy concerning what counts as disease.

Physical reductionists may dismiss my foregoing analysis, maintaining that advances in molecular biology will show that many behavioral abnormalities—now categorized as mental illnesses—will prove to be bona fide diseases displaying characteristic lesions on a subcellular level. I doubt it. But, supposing that that were to happen, the phenomena so identified would cease to be mental diseases and become instead infectious or neurological diseases—much as paresis and epilepsy ceased to be mental diseases once their pathoanatomical and pathophysiological nature became established.[43] If physicians, politicians, and people reject the scientific definition of disease, as they do in seemingly ever-increasing numbers, then medicine ceases to be a science and becomes, instead, part magic and religion, and part economics and politics.

3

CLINICAL MEDICINE
Diagnosis

Medicine is not a science. Nevertheless, the delivery of Western medicine depends totally on science and the scientific method.

Cecil Textbook of Medicine[1]

I learned very early the difference between knowing the name of something and knowing something.

Richard Feynman[2]

Perhaps no component of medical care is more important to subsequent care than establishing a diagnosis. From this first step decisions emerge about treatment, prognosis, and the use of health resources.

Frank Vinicor, M.D., Centers for Disease Control and Prevention[3]

Medical science and medical practice, like science and technology, are different but equally potent forces for making human life better or worse, depending on how they are used. The medical scientist—pathologist, microbiologist, biochemist, geneticist, molecular biologist, and so forth—deals with materials, such as bodies, body fluids, tissues, cells, microbes, and chemicals. The practicing physician, sometimes called "clinician," deals with *persons,* who may or may not be sick and with chemical, physical, psychological, and social methods for diagnosing, treating, and influencing persons called "patients."

"Pathology," states Alvan R. Feinstein, professor of medicine at Yale Medical School, "is not clinical medicine. The two domains are completely different in their sites, materials, methods of observation and interpretation, and imme-diate goals. . . . The necropsy is, and remains, the final, crucial, common path-way in 'disease.' . . . [It] is of fundamental importance and irreplaceable in medical science."[4]

By contrast, clinical medicine is based on the physician's observation of the patient, sometimes called "clinical observation." The term "clinic" comes from the Greek *klinikos*, meaning bed, and refers to the practice of the physician standing by the patient's bedside while teaching students about the patient's ailment. In contemporary use, the term "clinical" is gravely abused, as hype and honorific, to impart gravity and reality to the patient's nonexistent illness, for example, calling common unhappiness "clinical depression"; to confer an aura of medical competence on nonmedical personnel engaged in nonmedical activities, for example, calling psychologists who deal with people rather than animals "clinical psychologists"; or to suggest that drugs of dubious value have been scientifically validated as efficacious, for example, advertising herbal medicines as "clinically tested."

The modern physician engages in countless activities that have little or nothing to do with scientific or clinical medicine: He advertises diseases or drugs, gives advice on the radio and television or expert testimony in court, acts as an advocate for children, the poor, certain classes of patients, and so forth. Despite the economic, legal, or political context of these acts, the rheto-ric of diagnosis plays a paramount role in all of them.

DIAGNOSIS: NAMING DISEASE

Webster's defines diagnosis as "the art or act of identifying a disease from its signs and symptoms." According to the *Oxford English Dictionary* (OED), it is the "determination of the nature of a diseased condition; . . . also, the opinion (formally stated) resulting from such investigation."

The concept of diagnosis is contingent on the concept of disease. Diagnosis is the *name of a disease*, just as, say, violet is the name of a flower. For example, the term "diabetes" names a type of abnormal glucose metabolism. The disease qua somatic pathology is the abnormal metabolism; the diagnosis, "diabetes," is its name. Somatic pathology is diagnosed by finding physical abnormalities in bodies or body parts. Disease qua somatic pathology may be asymptomatic, and changing the classification of diseases (nosology) can change the name but not the reality of somatic pathology as disease. Diseases (lesions) are facts of na-ture, whereas diagnoses (words) are artifacts constructed by human beings. *If we fail to keep this simple distinction in mind, we forfeit the possibility of under-standing the uses and abuses of the term "diagnosis."*

Names, semanticists love to remind us, are not things. Manipulating things is difficult, sometimes impossible. Manipulating names is easy. We do it all the time. Violet may be the name of a flower, a color, a woman, or a street. Similarly, a disease-sounding term may be the name of a pathological lesion or bodily malfunction, or the name of the malfunction of a car, computer, or economic system, or the behavior of an individual or group. As I noted earlier, we cannot distinguish between the literal and metaphorical uses of the term "disease" unless we identify its root meaning, agree that *it* is the literal meaning of the word, and treat all other uses of it as figures of speech. In conformity with traditional practice, I take the root meaning of disease to be a *bodily lesion*, understood to include not only structural malfunctions but also deviations from normal physiology, such as elevated blood pressure or lowered white cell count. If we accept this definition, then the term "diagnosis," used *literally*, refers to and is the name of a disease, and used *metaphorically*, refers to and is the name of a nondisease.[5]

By identifying diagnosis as an *opinion*, the OED recognizes that it refers to a judgment. Clearly, physicians are not the only people who make disease judgments. The process of diagnosing disease typically starts with the patient: he has aches or pains, feels fatigued or feverish, and concludes that he is ill; sometimes he even names his illness. If the patient complains about his body, then, in a medical context, his complaint constitutes a *symptom*, a medical-sounding word that misleadingly implies that his experience is a manifestation of a disease. *Webster's* defines symptom as "subjective evidence of disease or physical disturbance *observed by the patient*" (emphasis added). In other words, a symptom may or may not indicate the presence of disease.

The accuracy of the clinical diagnosis rests heavily on the kinds of information on which it is based, the methods used to obtain it, and the observer's interpretation of it. It may be based solely on the patient's medical history and complaints or may, in addition, take into account objective, pathological data, such as the examination of a biopsy specimen and laboratory tests. In contrast, the pathological diagnosis is based almost entirely on objective evidence, and may, accordingly, be based on histological, morphological, chemical, serological, and other technical information.

Historically, scientific medicine is based on the postmortem examination of the body. Recalling his early work as a *neurologist*, Freud proudly reminisced: "The fame of my diagnoses and *their post-mortem confirmation* brought me an influx of American physicians, to whom I lectured upon the patients in my department in a sort of pidgin-English."[6] In scientific medicine, the pathological diagnosis always trumps the clinical diagnosis.

The use of diagnostic terms becomes problematic when the conditions they name are not diseases but merely subjective, unverifiable complaints, referable to an individual's body, behaviors, or thoughts (communications). Psychopathology is diagnosed by finding unwanted behaviors in persons or by attributing such behaviors to them. For example, the term "kleptomania" is both a phenomenon and a name; diagnosis and disease are one and the same. Once "named," the diagnosis of a mental illness validates its own disease status. Psychopathology, unlike organic pathology, can change with the nosology—changing the name can convert disease into nondisease and vice versa (for example, homosexuality into civil right, smoking into nicotine dependence). Mental diseases are, *a fortiori*, diagnoses, not diseases.[7]

Diagnoses Are Not Diseases

The differences between disease and diagnosis are clear and uncontroversial. They may be summarized as follows:

- Disease is a *fact*; diagnosis is an *opinion*. Diseases are *discovered;* diagnoses are *created.* Diseases cannot be manufactured, but diagnoses can be.

- Diabetes is a disease, regardless of whether anyone recognizes or interprets it as such. It is a biologically constructed disease. Depression is a diagnosis, recognized as a disease only if it is authoritatively interpreted as such. It is a "socially constructed" disease.

- The concept of disease belongs in the realm of biology. Old diseases disappear (smallpox) and new diseases appear (AIDS) because of changes in the physical/material world. The concept of diagnosis belongs in the realm of history. Old diagnoses may disappear (dropsy) and new diagnoses appear (congestive heart failure) because of changes in the social and technical world.

Notwithstanding the distinctions between disease and diagnosis, the public, science writers, and even some leading physicians persistently conflate and confuse the two concepts. "Definitions of illness do not belong solely to the white-coated realm of pure science," asserts a popular science writer.[8] "Should the patient's experience or the doctor's test define the disease? . . . Should cancer be defined and diagnosed by pathologists or others?" asks Robert A. Aronowitz, professor of medicine at the Robert Wood Johnson Medical School, New Jersey.[9]

The results of such dumbing down of the discourse about disease and diagnosis are all around us. Using a poll surveying the nation's health, *Parade* magazine concluded that depression is "the third most common *disease* reported by our survey respondents." Yet when the respondents were asked, "What is your greatest personal health concern for the future?," they did not even mention depression. They were concerned about cancer and heart disease.[10] Even though people have accepted the categorization of depression as a disease, they are not afraid of getting depression because they intuitively recognize that it is a personal problem, not a disease; but they are afraid of getting cancer and heart disease because they know these are diseases—true medical problems—not just names.

A reporter for *Forbes* writes: "All of a sudden there are pharmacological solutions to conditions from shyness to erectile dysfunction that drugmakers tell us are no longer facts of life but diseases."[11] Drugmakers don't make diagnoses; doctors do. Another reporter scoffs at the diagnosis of "social phobia"—a.k.a shyness—but is confident that "the majority of conditions" listed in the American Psychiatric Association's *Diagnostic and Statistical Manual of Mental Disorders (DSM-IV)* are diseases.[12] But if this diagnosis does not name a *real disease*, what makes him so sure that others do?

While seemingly critical of the psychiatric enterprise, such reports strengthen and support it.[13] Objecting to a particular psychiatric diagnosis—like objecting to a particular psychiatric treatment, such as drugs or electroshock therapy—implies that only the particular diagnosis or treatment in question is invalid and that all the others are valid. The truth is that no psychiatric diagnosis—not merely this or that one—names a condition that meets the classic pathological criterion of disease.

Regarding the fatuous notion that "definitions of illness do not belong solely to the white-coated realm of pure science," let me restate that, because we have free speech, anyone can define any term. However, when a person calls a dolphin a fish, we don't affirm his right to define what counts as a fish, but dismiss his definition as ill-informed. Similarly, anyone can define disease, but the scientific definition of the concept of disease belongs to medical scientists, just as the scientific definition of the concept of the electron belongs to physicists.

Science writers and the public overlook or ignore that patients, physicians, relatives, insurance companies, pharmaceutical manufacturers, and the state have different interests in what *ought to count* as a (diagnosable and/or treatable) disease. Practicing physicians want to treat patients rationally, relieve their complaints, and collect a satisfactory fee for their services. Patients want relief from illness and suffering. Others—so-called third parties (relatives, insurance companies, the state)—want many different outcomes, such as saving the patient's life, providing an expensive treatment for him, letting him die, securing or refusing reimbursement for the cost of treatment, and so forth. The differences that divide these parties *are matters of self-interest, not matters of fact or reasoning*.

The confusion of diagnosis with disease is not an occasional, innocent error. If it were, it would have been corrected long ago. Rather, it is a systematic and

Table 1
Disease, Patient, and the Medical-Social Situation

Disease	Patient	Medical Situation: Physician-Patient Relationship (If Any)
+	+	The scientifically sick person who seeks medical help: the standard model of the consenting patient
+	-	The scientifically sick person who does not seek medical help: the standard model of the sick nonpatient; e.g., denial of illness or rejection of medical treatment on religious or other grounds
-	+	The well person who seeks medical help: the standard model of the "malingerer," "hypochondriac," etc.; the well person who seeks a "regular checkup" as a preventive measure; the "worried well"
-	-	The well person who does not seek medical help: the standard model of the healthy nonpatient

Source: Adapted from T. Szasz, *Insanity: The Idea and Its Consequences*, p. 34.

strategic error, a tactical misuse of language that serves the pharmacratic ideology. Calling a personal problem or interpersonal conflict a disease enlarges the power of the classifier, as the following example illustrates: "BOSTON (AP)—A convicted killer who says he is a woman trapped in a man's body has filed a federal lawsuit to force the State to pay for a sex change. Robert Kosilek, who is serving a life sentence for killing his wife in 1990, claims it is cruel and unusual punishment to prevent him from becoming a woman."[14]

Conflating disease and diagnosis is useful to anyone who, for whatever reason, wants to obscure the distinctions between *having a disease (lesion)* and *being a patient (social role)*. Ignoring or rejecting this distinction allows us to treat patients as if they were sick, to treat sick persons as if they were patients, and to continue the intellectually barren but economically and professionally rewarding debate about the connections between diagnoses and treatments—especially about the efficacy or lack thereof of treating patients without bodily diseases (sometimes even without their consent) with drugs, electricity, neurosurgery, psychotherapy, and placebos. (See Table 1.)

The therapeutic implications of the foregoing distinctions may be schematically summarized, as follows:

- If the physician addresses disease as somatic pathology, the goal of treatment is ameliorating or curing the disease that causes the patient's symptoms/suffering. The sole criterion for assessing the scientific efficacy of the intervention is the appropriate response of the somatic-pathological processes, measured by objective methods. The patient's improved sense of well-being is a dividend paid by this investment. (Treatment aimed at making the patient feel better, without beneficially impinging on the disease process, is called "palliative" or "symptomatic").

- If the physician addresses disease as psychopathology, the goal of treatment and the criterion for its efficacy depend on whether the subject is a voluntary or involuntary patient.

  - If the subject is a voluntary patient, the goal of treatment is to make him feel better. The main criterion for assessing the efficacy of the intervention is the patient's opinion.

  - If the subject is an involuntary patient, the direct or primary goal of treatment (civil commitment and some other intervention) is to make others feel better (about the patient or about being relieved of him). The sole criterion for assessing the efficacy of the intervention is the opinion of others (judges, psychiatrists, relatives). The patient's opinion is irrelevant.

- If the individual medicates himself (with legal or illegal drugs) or the physician medicates the patient with a placebo, the goal of treatment is to make oneself or the patient feel better. The sole criterion for assessing the efficacy of the intervention is the subjective response of the self/patient.

My observation about the involuntary patient requires a further comment. Psychiatrists not only *define* what they consider unwanted behaviors as diseases, for example, self-abuse and homosexuality in the past, drug abuse and homophobia today; they also *define* what they consider improved behaviors—produced, for example, by lobotomy, electroshock, or psychotropic drugs—as the results of treatments. In 1948 Paul Hoch (1902–1964), professor of psychiatry at Columbia University and the Commissioner of Mental Hygiene for New York State, explained the therapeutic effectiveness of physical treatments of mental illnesses as follows: "This brings us for a moment to a discussion of the brain damage produced by electroshock. . . . Is a certain amount of brain damage not necessary in this type of treatment? Frontal lobotomy indicates that improvement takes place by a definite damage of certain parts of the brain."[15]

Unless we acknowledge the identity of the agents responsible for defining what counts as disease/treatment, we deceive others as well as ourselves about the differences not only between disease and diagnosis, but also between literal (somatic) treatments (influencing the body) and metaphorical (mental) treatments (influencing the person). The very existence of the Office of Alternative

Medicine at the NIH—an agency ostensibly dedicated to determining the scientific effectiveness, if any, of medical treatments—is evidence that the term "treatment" may or may not refer to a procedure scientifically demonstrated to be effective. If alternative medicine is valid, it belongs to mainstream medicine; if it is not valid, it is quackery. There is no alternative astronomy, chemistry, or physics. The term "alternative medicine" is tacit acknowledgment that certain medical practices are scientifically invalid, albeit some doctors and patients may find them useful.

THE CORRUPTION OF MEDICINE

People who do not feel well often view the presumed cause of their malaise as a disease. As noted earlier, professionals and lay persons often classify things differently. The zoologist calls a dolphin a mammal, whereas a layman may call it a fish. The logic is impeccable. Fishes are aquatic animals, the dolphin is an aquatic animal, therefore the dolphin is a fish.[16] Similarly, lay persons, especially when they do not feel well and regard themselves as patients, often believe, or even insist, that certain nondiseases are diseases. They fail to distinguish diseases from nondiseases for the same reason that they fail to distinguish dolphins from fishes, namely, because making such a distinction requires specialized knowledge.

However, physicians, especially the editors of prestigious medical journals and experts in various medical specialties, know better. Why, then, do they also frequently fail to distinguish diagnoses from diseases and give disease names to conditions that lack any of the criteria of disease? It is unseemly to attribute base motives to persons with whom one disagrees and I will therefore not answer the question. Suffice it to say that the practice of attributing disease status to nondiseases is now so common even among medical elites that it is fair to conclude that the medical profession is guilty, beyond a reasonable doubt, of corrupting its own concept of disease.

Debasing Diagnoses: Giving Disease Names to Nondiseases

Rulers seeking to enlarge their political power always needed more money than they had—for paying mercenaries to fight for them and for making their supporters dependent on their largesse. As long as money was gold coin, the rulers' typical tactic—second only to robbing enemies or scapegoats—was debasing the currency by issuing coin consisting partly or wholly of metals less precious than gold. (I return to this subject in more detail later in this chapter.) For example, Philip IV (1268 [1285]–1314)—King of France, better known as Philip Le Bel or the Fair because of his good looks—was nicknamed "the counterfeiter," because he relentlessly debased the coin.[17] He also relentlessly "taxed" and eventually expropriated the Jews.[18] (This tactic—stigmatizing scapegoats as irredeemably vile and filthy rich to boot, and exploiting them as a source of revenue—was popular among Christian monarchs in the Middle Ages and is now employed by the therapeutic state against tobacco companies.)

The medical profession has engaged in a similar process, debasing diagnosis by counting certain nondiseases (behaviors) as diseases. Initially confined largely to psychiatry, since the end of World War II the process has spread to other areas of medicine and has greatly accelerated as well. Herewith an example.

In its January 13, 2000 issue, the *New England Journal of Medicine* published a "Special Article" entitled "Mass Psychogenic Illness Attributed to Toxic Exposure at a High School." The report was prepared by eight authors, bore the imprimatur of the Centers for Disease Control and Prevention and Vanderbilt University Medical School, and was accompanied by an editorial that reemphasized the importance of the subject and the authors' conclusions.[19] Before commenting on the report, I want to note that the very term "psychogenic illness" is a misnomer: The term "psychogenic" is a euphemism for "self-inflicted" or "self-caused"; the correct adjective ought to be "autogenic" or "egogenic." The phenomenon so qualified is *caused* by the self, not the soul, the spirit, the mind, or the brain—and it is not an illness.

The report is an account of a high school teacher noticing "a 'gasoline-like' smell in her classroom," after which "she had a headache, nausea, shortness of breath, and dizziness. The school was evacuated, and 80 students and 19 staff members went to the emergency room at the local hospital; 38 persons were hospitalized overnight. Five days later, after the school had reopened, another 71 persons went to the emergency room."[20] The subjects as well as their physical environment were studied extensively and it was concluded that the subjects' complaints could not be attributed to an environmental cause. The authors' diagnosis was "epidemic hysteria, also referred to as mass psychogenic or sociogenic illness."

The editorial accompanying the report refers to the students' and teachers' imitating each other's behavior as a "rapid outbreak of illness" and concludes: "Psychogenic symptoms are physiologic experiences that are based on identifiable physiologic processes that cause pain and suffering."[21] This interpretation precludes the possibility of distinguishing phenomena properly classified as illnesses (formerly validated as "organic" or "bodily") from phenomena properly classified as not illnesses (formerly invalidated as "functional" or "mental").[22]

In my view, the most important issue discussed by Jones and colleagues and the editorial is not psychogenic illness, but the *demarcation between illness and nonillness*. There is no verifiable difference between a "psychogenic" and an "organic" symptom (unless the latter term is used incorrectly, in lieu of "sign").

Symptoms are complaints, always "real" to the complainant. Many complaints that meet the authors' definition of psychogenic symptom—for example, unrelieved sexual excitement or suppressed rage provoked by a gratuitous insult—do not qualify as illnesses, unless every unwanted experience be regarded as an illness.

Creating a taxonomic category—say, "money," "fish," or "illness"—implies a commitment to excluding items that do not belong in it, especially deliberate imitations. Counterfeit is not money, dolphins are not fish, and imaginary illnesses are not diseases. The fact that "psychogenic illnesses" seem real to patients as well as doctors, or that both want to treat them as if they were illnesses, is irrelevant to this conclusion.[23]

Calling complaints about the body "illnesses," despite the absence of objective evidence of illness, is a violation of elementary rules of logic, an offense against scientific medicine, and an act of medical hubris.[24] Nevertheless, the exigencies and pressures of medical practice pose an unremitting temptation to fudge the boundaries between *symptom and sign, complaint and lesion, illness and nonillness.* For many practicing physicians, in some specialties more than in others, *not* fudging the boundaries would be tantamount to professional suicide.

Practicing physicians, especially family doctors, must, at least provisionally, accept their patient's *complaints* of pain, malaise, fatigue, and insomnia at face value, as if they were the symptoms of disease.[25] Worse, they are under duress to *prescribe* chemically active drugs for them, regardless of whether the patients have demonstrable diseases or, if they have such diseases, whether the prescribed treatment is effective. Trying to make patients believe that "something is being done" for them, physicians feel compelled not only to treat many nondiseases as if they were diseases, but to justify doing so by medicalizing the patients' complaints and publishing pseudoscientific accounts of their ailments in medical journals.

The term "functional somatic syndrome" *sounds* like the name of a disease, but it is not a disease. Arthur J. Barsky and Jonathan F. Borus—the authors of a major review-article of this "illness" in the *Annals of Internal Medicine,* the official journal of the American College of Physicians—recognize that the phenomena they describe are not genuine diseases. Nevertheless, they give the patients' complaints disease names, discuss their complaints as if they were diseases, and offer what they regard as medical treatments for them.[26]

"The term *functional somatic syndrome,*" Barsky and Borus explain, "refers to several related syndromes that are characterized more by symptoms, suffering, and disability than by disease-specific, demonstrable abnormalities of structure and function."[27] What are some "functional somatic syndromes?" Multiple chemical sensitivity, chronic whiplash, the side effects of silicone breast implants, candidiasis hypersensitivity, and hypoglycemia. Formerly popular but now increasingly passé "functional somatic syndromes" are symptoms attributed to chronic carbon monoxide poisoning, exposure to video display terminals, carbonless copy paper, and weak electromagnetic fields.[28]

People eager to play the sick role seek medical services for, and other benefits from, being sick and disabled; hence, they may be of great economic value to doctors and lawyers. Consider how Barsky and Borus describe the clients: "Physicians in many medical specialties are increasingly confronted by patients who have *disabling*, medically unexplained, *somatic symptoms* and who have already arrived at a diagnostic label for their *illness*."[29] The term "somatic symptom" is medical jargon for complaint about the body. Its use implies that the problem at hand is medical, an assumption inconsistent with the authors' subsequent remarks: "The functional somatic syndromes have acquired major sociocultural and political dimensions. Their definitive status in public consciousness and popular discourse contrasts markedly with their still uncertain scientific and biomedical status. Patients with these syndromes often have very explicit disease attributions for their symptoms, and they resist information that contradicts these attributions." In other words, the patient believes he has a disease even though he has no identifiable disease. It is not clear why Barsky and Borus expect the patients to accept information contrary to their beliefs, especially when physicians ratify the patients' false beliefs: They give the patients' nondiseases disease names and attribute them to nonexistent infectious agents which they treat as if they were real.

Stephen E. Ross, also writing in the *Annals of Internal Medicine*, explains: "Memes are infectious agents in psychosomatic illness." What is a meme? It is "a virulent idea . . . [that] can be found at the core of these diverse disorders . . . such disease conceptions, which I [Ross] term *psychosomatic memes*, act as transmissible templates."[30] If we let doctors make up diagnoses and infectious agents out of whole cloth, why not let patients make up diseases out of symptoms?

Let us be honest: Classifying nondiseases as diseases serves the economic, existential, and professional interest of the classifiers and is, to boot, socially expected of them. For the vast majority of health-care professionals—especially the legions of psychologists, social workers, grief counselors, drug abuse specialists, and other practitioners of existential cannibalism—it would be professional suicide to categorize nondiseases correctly: their every instinct of self-interest opposes such truth telling. After incessantly inflating the concept of illness, medical professionals and the media have, in effect, lost their ability *to call a spade a spade and a heart a nonspade.* Confronted with sufficient pressure from individuals, institutions, and the state, they are too confused or too timid to call phenomena that lack the requisite features of diseases, "nondiseases."

Although a behavior may be the cause of a disease, and a complaint may be a consequence of disease, *neither a behavior nor a complaint is, by itself, a disease.*

Boxing may cause disease but is not a disease. Pain may be a consequence of disease, but is not a disease. No wonder that mental health professionals, eager to legitimize their activities as *medical*, explicitly assert the opposite: "Functional impairment or *disability, not the presence of a lesion*, is the essential element in the *medical* concept of disease."[31] This is false. But increasingly fewer people realize that it is false. Let us see why this is so.

DISEASE IS TO DIAGNOSIS AS GOLD IS TO MONEY

To understand the abuses of a system of classification, we must first understand its uses. As the periodic table was not created for commercial purposes, so classic medical nosology was not created for therapeutic purposes. I am pointing here to an aspect of the distinction between science and technology, theory and application—a distinction especially decisive in the early stages of science. As a rule, theory comes first, applications follow later. Michael Faraday (1791–1867) may have known more about electricity than Thomas Edison (1847–1931), but he never saw an electric light bulb. A similar lag in applying medical science to medical treatment characterizes the history of medicine.

To recreate the scene of late-nineteenth-century medicine, it is necessary to place its practice in its proper political-economic context. Prior to World War I, medical practice was a personal service, distributed by physicians, hospitals, and pharmaceutical companies for money, to those who could pay for it, and as a charity to those who could not. The physician's income depended solely on the patient's ability and willingness to pay for the services he wanted; it was, for all practical purposes, unrelated to the diagnosis the doctor attached to his disease. Like other personal services in a capitalist society, the distribution of medical care was want-based, "rationed" by the market. Patients willing to pay market prices could receive all the care they wanted, from doctors, nurses, pharmacists, hospitals, sanatoria, spas, and similar establishments, regardless of whether they were sick or not, or whether the service was medically indicated or not. Residing in a hospital in those days was more like staying in a resort today than it is like being hospitalized today. The providers of medical services did not ask the would-be patient whether he *needed* medical services, just as the providers of resort services do not ask the would-be tourist whether he *needs* a vacation.

If a third party joins a two-person game, its rules ipso facto are altered. If an insurance company or the state becomes an active participant in the business of defining what counts as medical care as well as in paying for and distributing the service, the nature of medical practice undergoes a process of metamorphosis: the economics of medicine, the power relations between doctor and patient, and the very meaning and implications of key terms all change. This is familiar territory. "He who pays the piper calls the tune." Troy Duster, professor of sociology at the University of California, in Berkeley, phrases it more professionally: "Once the third party steps in to pay the physician for delivering health-care to the patient, the interests of the third party will typically supersede those of the patient."[32] Economists recognize that once people cease having to pay for the medical services they want, the demand for the services skyrockets. It is odd, then, that economists and health-care policy experts refuse to recognize that once the physician ceases to be paid directly by his patient for the services he *wants*, and is instead paid by others to deliver services the patient ostensibly *needs, the physician's propensity to make certain diagnoses or discover new diseases by creating disease names skyrockets*. It is even odder that the experts stubbornly deny that, in the West, the first physicians paid for their services by the state rather than their patients were the mad-doctors, now called "psychiatrists"; that psychiatrists were the first manufacturers of diagnoses masquerading as diseases; and that, ever since, psychiatrists have been the leading producers of the conceptually and economically important commodity we call "mental illnesses."

To be sure, the psychiatrist is not the only physician who is an agent of the state rather than of the patient. The military physician serves the interests of the military; the public health physician, the interests of the public; and so forth. However, the public health physician's work was based on the application of scientific criteria to disease control: he was concerned primarily with sanitation and the control of infectious diseases; hence, he had no economic or professional interest in manufacturing new diagnoses/diseases. This is no longer true. The Surgeon General is now a political appointee, a medical hack whose job is to serve his political masters.

The Political Economy of Diagnosis

As expenditures on health-care services shift from the citizen to the state, political-economic forces determine how and how much of the taxpayer's money is spent on such services. Various government agencies are always in competition for the state's limited resources. This stimulates a demand, both private and public, that the system be protected from "exploitation by special interest groups," especially patients and doctors, and leads to the creation of new bureaucratic organizations, charged with preventing patients from receiving "medically unnecessary" services, and physicians from receiving payment for such services.

During the second half of the twentieth century, the practice of Western medicine was transformed from a system rationed mainly by the market to a system controlled mainly by bureaucratic rules and regulations with diagnoses used to rationalize the distribution of services. Unlike in England and Europe, in the United States this transformation was accompanied by celebratory lip service to the marvels of the free market, blinding most Americans to the fact that the free market in drugs as well as in medical services had, for some time, been barred and even criminalized. People interested in taking drugs, but prevented from buying them on the open market by prescription laws, must acquire diagnoses to justify being prescribed and dispensed such drugs. Pharmaceutical manufacturers eager to sell drugs to eager buyers, but prevented by the same laws from selling them directly to the public, need physicians to attach appropriate diagnoses to patients, so that the patients can obtain the drugs they want. Manufacturing medical diagnoses helps patients, physicians, and pharmaceutical manufacturers to achieve these goals. Pharmaceutical companies pressuring patients to "consult your doctor" and ask for a specific drug—in a barrage of advertising aimed directly at the public, nurturing the illusion that people can control their health care—completes the cycle of nonscientific approach to diagnosis and treatment.

Everything that has a function can fail to work properly or work at all. If the item that fails is manmade—for example, an electric switch—we say it malfunctions. However, if the item that fails is a person or a particular aspect of personal performance—such as sexual functioning—then we say that the person suffers from a "dysfunction." *Voilà*, a new malady has been created.

This foolishness is accepted as science by both American medicine and American law. The media and the people love the resulting spectacle. For a spectacle it is, as illustrated by a story titled "Bad News in the Bedroom," from *Newsweek*. "*Everyone* is at risk of sexual dysfunction, sooner or later," explained sociologist Edward O. Laumann, in the *Journal of the American Medical Association*.[33] Laumann, *mirabile dictu*, was a paid consultant to Pfizer, manufacturer of Viagra.

Everyone with a modicum of medical knowledge knows that one of the common consequences of removing a man's cancerous prostate is that many of the nerves supplying the genital area may be severed, making it impossible for the subject to have an erection. Former senator and former presidential candidate Bob Dole advertises "courage" and Viagra in magazines and on television, his credential being that he has "erectile dysfunction," or "ED." Until recently, the condition from which Mr. Dole suffers was considered a sequela of total prostatectomy, not a distinct and separate disease.

What happened to Mr. Dole after he had prostate surgery is similar to what happened to President Franklin D. Roosevelt after he had polio. Each suffered from an interruption of nerve conduction, resulting in a condition called "paralysis." Roosevelt did not have "walking dysfunction"; he was paralyzed. Dole does not have "sexual dysfunction"; he is impotent. The rhetoric he spouts is not medical science, it is junk science or pseudoscience, the same junk science that gives us "behavioral dysfunctions," "emotional dysfunctions," "mood dysfunctions," and so forth. Each dysfunction, of course, is said to be "treatable," as if calling a condition "treatable" proved that "it" is a disease.

Like much mischief in medicine, the notion that we can infer disease from "treatability" was created by psychiatrists. Yet, a famous psychiatrist—Manfred Bleuler (1903–1994), the son of the famed psychiatrist Eugen Bleuler (1857–1939), a professor of psychiatry at the University of Zurich and director of the Burgholzli mental hospital—warned: "After the introduction of sleep therapy, and cardiazole-, insulin-, and electroshock therapies for schizophrenics, the argument was often raised that the discovery of a specific physical therapy indicated a specific physical disease. Subsequent experience effectively refuted such assumptions."[34] The assumption is, a priori, fallacious.

In the old system of distributing health care, the physician was a private entrepreneur: the most costly treatments went to those persons who had the most money. In the new system, the physician is in effect an agent of the state (or some other third party, directly or indirectly regulated by the state): the most costly medical care is delivered to those patients whose diagnoses justify the most costly or most reimbursable treatments. In the capitalist system, the financially most successful physicians are those with the wealthiest patients; a hundred years ago, unscrupulous physicians who catered to the whims of the rich made more money than did conscientious physicians who cared for the ills of ordinary people and refrained from using popular but harmful medical interventions. In the contemporary American-statist system, the financially most successful physicians are those who cease to practice medicine and instead become medical entrepreneurs. Among those who stay in medicine, the financially best rewarded physicians are those with the most reimbursable procedures for sale: oncologists treating hopelessly ill cancer patients are among the highest earners in the profession, while pediatricians averting preventable diseases in healthy children with the greatest life expectancy are among the lowest.

Because the need for medical services and the compensation physicians receive for such services are often not medically determined at all, neither the private-capitalist nor the public-statist system is or can be "fair" or "rational." Treatment of erectile dysfunction in a 70-year-old man is reimbursed by Medicare, but treatment of infertility in a 30-year-old woman is not reimbursed by medical insurance. Wealthy persons and powerful politicians can buy any medical service they want, regardless of what society they live in, whether or not they "need" the services. The opposite is true for poor and powerless persons. Capitalist medicine favors the rich in obvious ways. Socialist medicine penalizes the poor less obviously but perhaps even more seriously.

DIAGNOSIS AND THE ECONOMICS OF HEALTH CARE

Goods and services may be distributed according to what people want and are able to afford, or, if they lack financial resources, according to what they need and receive from a benefactor, such as a parent, charitable institution, or the state.[35] As we shift from a want-based to a need-based system of receiving medical services and drugs, it is easy to reify diagnosis and lose sight of the fact that treatment is a medical service that *people* receive or reject, not something that diagnoses receive or reject. A headline in the *New York Times*, "Using Gene Testing to Decide a Patient's Treatment," illustrates this misconception.[36] A diagnostic test *informs* the physician and the patient about a particular aspect of the patient's bodily functioning. The test cannot and does not *decide* on the treatment.

In a want-based system of health care, adults receive what they want, pay for, and someone is willing to sell. (Infants and other dependents receive what they need, as determined by their caretaker.) "Money," quipped George Bernard Shaw, "enables us to get what we want instead of what other people think we want."[37] With respect to health care services, Shaw's dictum may be rephrased as follows: "Money enables us to get the medical care we want instead of the care other people think we *need because of our medical condition*."

Until World War II, the delivery and cost of most medical care in the United States was want-based—capitalist, individualist, and (relatively) free of interference by the state or insurance companies. Persons unable to pay for medical services received care gratis, as charity; the delivery of such services was controlled by persons in charge of particular charitable organizations and by physicians. Patients had virtually no say in the matter, save for being free to reject charitable medical care (excepting psychiatric care). The delivery of over-the-counter drugs and other commodities that have far-reaching effects on health—such as food, housing, and recreation—is still essentially want-based.

By contrast, the delivery of most medical care in the United States is now need-based—bureaucratic-statist, paid, partly or entirely, by Medicare, Medicaid, or so-called private health insurance. Access to, and reimbursement for, medical services is premised on the assumptions that its proper distribution is the duty of the state or other third party; HMOs should approve and insurance companies should pay only for the treatment of conditions they regard as diseases and only if treated by methods they approve; and physicians should treat patients not according to their own judgment, subject to the patient's consent, but according to criteria determined by the medical profession and the HMO or insurance company. The result is twofold: both patient and physician lose control over the doctor-patient relationship, and the physician's diagnosis is transformed from a descriptive term identifying the patient's disease to a strategic and justificatory term aimed at supporting a claim for delivering a treatment and receiving payment for it. To receive reimbursement for his services, the physician thus gives his patient a diagnosis, whether or not he has a disease; and to justify giving the patient a treatment for which payment is explicitly excluded by his insurance, and nevertheless receive payment for it, the physician gives him a false diagnosis. An American version of this scheme is known as the DRG system, that is, medical reimbursement based on a set of diagnostic criteria called "diagnosis-related groups" (DRGs). Note that this scheme makes it seem as if medical services were delivered to diagnoses instead of to *people*.

Diagnosing for Dollars: DRGs

The original aim of DRGs, adopted in 1967 by the Health Care Finance Administration (an agency of the federal government), was to control the costs of treating hospitalized patients under the Medicare system.[38] "Each DRG takes the principal diagnosis or procedure responsible for a patient's admission, and is given a corresponding cost weighting. This weight is applied according to a formula to determine the amount that should be paid to an institution for a patient with a particular DRG."[39] Soon, the method was applied to outpatients covered by Medicare and Medicaid as well as by private health insurance.

In theory, DRGs relate a patient's diagnosis to the cost of his treatment.[40] In practice, DRGs are an attempt to substitute ostensibly objective measures of the cost of various medical services (estimated by the government-as-payer), for the subjective value persons-as-patients place on various medical services (measured by how much of their own money individuals are willing to spend for them). Once governments decide that it is their duty to provide health care services for people, recourse to some mechanism to determine "medical need" and "effective treatment" "becomes a practical necessity: Health-care bureaucrats, economists, and statisticians promptly rise to the occasion and develop "fair" and "equitable" schedules of reimbursement. (Private health insurance companies follow their lead.) Thus begins the game in which hospitals and physicians are the principal players: Winning means maximizing reimbursement by placing every patient into the most financially favorable diagnostic category.

Unfortunately, the attempt to relate the value/cost of medical services (reimbursement) to the names of diseases (diagnoses) rests on three hugely erroneous assumptions: (1) that the relief of illness is a scientific-technical matter, best determined by medical experts; (2) that the diagnoses used by the system name objectively identifiable (literal) diseases; and (3) that pegging payment to physicians to the diagnoses they make does not affect their diagnostic behavior.

It defies common sense and everyday experience to believe that, for the same diagnosis/disease, people—whether princes or paupers, VIPs (very important persons) or VUPs (very unimportant persons)—need, and ought to receive, the same treatment. In real life, the powerful and the powerless are bound to be offered different treatment options for the same diagnosis/disease; moreover, even if offered the same options, each might make different choices, reflecting their particular needs and values. The same goes for people with different temperaments and values. Although the hypochondriac and the stoic may suffer from the same disease, the former values medical services more highly than the latter and seeks more of them.[41] Medical bureaucrats confuse not only diagnoses with diseases, but also objective disease entities with peoples' subjective judgments regarding the need for and value of their treatment. In the case of psychiatric diagnoses—for example, 312.33 Pyromania, 312.31 Pathological Gambling, 313.81 Oppositional Defiant Disorder, 300.7 Body Dysmorphic Disorder, and 307.42 Primary Insomnia—it is plainly false that the diagnostic terms name objectively identifiable diseases.[42]

Actually, the DRGs and *DSMs* are parasitic on one another: the *Diagnostic and Statistical Manuals* feed the diagnosis-related groups with diagnoses authenticated as diseases by the medical profession and the government, and the DRGs in turn revalidate the diagnoses in the *DSMs* as the names of bona fide diseases. The authors of *DSM-IV* deny this, declaring: "*DSM-IV* is a classification of mental disorders that was developed for use in clinical, educational, and research settings."[43] Not true. The diagnoses of most mental diseases are *used to justify* the psychiatrist's obligation to commit patients or his need to prescribe drugs and other so-called treatments for them, collecting third-party payments for their treatment, and assisting lawyers engaged in civil and criminal litigation making use of psychiatric concepts and interventions.

Although scaling payment for medical services to DRGs rests on fundamentally faulty assumptions—notably, the physician is not paid for ruling out a particular disease, which is a very important medical service—the DRG system has become an important element in the new medical discipline called "medical informatics." Enrico Coiera, the author of a basic text in the field, explains: "If physiology literally means 'the logic of life,' and pathology is 'the logic of disease,' then *medical informatics is the logic of health care*. . . . It is likely that in the next century, the study of informatics will become as fundamental to the practice of medicine as anatomy has been to the last."[44] This is nothing less than an admission that, henceforth, *the diagnosis of the bureaucrat replaces the determination of the pathologist as the criterion for what counts as disease—for the purpose of allocating care to patients and paying physicians, hospitals, therapists, drug companies, and others for their services.*

The once-revered clinical-pathological conference—clinical medicine's sacred ritual—has thus been demoted to an academic exercise. Although still valued for checking the clinical diagnosis against the pathological diagnosis, it is not where the action, let alone the money, is. The money is in diagnosing for dollars, not in diagnosing for accuracy. Coiera recognizes that DRG diagnoses and traditional diagnoses serve different purposes and comments: "In medicine, one way to deal with this lack of clarity is to *create artificial definitions of disease concepts with a purpose in mind.* . . . A general purpose terminology will always fail to meet many of the specific needs of different situations."[45] This is a truism habitually neglected in medicine, especially psychiatry. Obviously, different criteria of disease and diagnosis are needed to rationalize removing a person's inflamed appendix with his consent, justify depriving an innocent person of liberty by incarcerating him in a mental hospital, and assigning economic value to a particular diagnostic or therapeutic intervention.[46]

Making reimbursement for treatment dependent on diagnosis creates a host of ethical and social problems. "The greatest danger with DRGs," observes a physician, "may result from linking monetary gain to the classification system, an idea supported by the current literature."[47] Another physician puts it more bluntly: "The sicker *you make* a patient look, the more money you get."[48] Physicians rationalize the chicanery by telling themselves that everyone "has something" that can be diagnosed and joke about scattering "confetti diagnoses" across billings forms.

As we might expect, diagnoses are most often and most obviously constructed and deconstructed in response to nonmedical considerations in situations when the health/disease issue pertains to VIPs in the public eye, and when the alleged disease affects personal—sexual or mental—functioning. Most people recognize the politically motivated fabrications and falsifications of the diagnoses of presidents such as Franklin D. Roosevelt and John F. Kennedy. However, they do not recognize the legally motivated fabrications and falsifications of the diagnoses of criminals, such as John W. Hinckley, Jr. and Theodore Kaczynski.

The economically motivated fabrications and falsifications of diagnoses receive the most media attention. There is steady stream of reports in newspapers and magazines about what doctors are "forced" to do to get paid for their services. For example, "The visit doesn't get paid if [the family physician] write[s] down depression. Because that's a psychiatric diagnosis. However the doctor knows that if she writes down the diagnosis 'fatigue' instead, she can still see those patients . . . and prescribe an antidepressant like Zoloft."[49]

In billing for hospital costs, the construction of diagnoses is no longer in the hands of physicians at all. Instead, the job is delegated to medical records personnel assisted by so-called code consultants, whose task is to help "upcode" diagnoses. The term refers to the practice of upgrading the seriousness of an illness by filing Medicare bills under the DRG code that carries the highest reimbursement. A *Wall Street Journal* article cites the example of a DRG consultant upcoding from "simple pneumonia" (worth $2,991) to "pneumonia, complications" (worth $4,462).[50] According to the *Journal,* the practice is endemic in the industry.

Diagnosing for Compassion: Medical Ethics in Action

Making payment for medical services dependent on diagnoses leads many physicians to "game" the system. From a story in *U.S. News & World Report*, titled "Is Your Doctor Lying for You?," we learn that because some insurance plans do not cover treatment for depression, Daniel Sulmasy, chair of the department of ethics at St. Vincent's Hospital and Medical Center in New York, writes down a code for " 'sleep disorder' if a depressed person is having trouble sleeping. . . . Then he can prescribe a medication, like Paxil." [51] Of course, the physician could prescribe Paxil even if he coded for depression, except in that case the patient would have to pay for the drug.

This is not a dilemma about ethics, it is a dilemma about money. Miscoding from a noninsured diagnosis to an insured diagnosis is simply cheating the insurance company and rationalizing this as helping the patient. "That doctors regularly fudge on health-insurance forms," writes a reporter for *Time* magazine, "is one of the dirty little secrets of American medicine. . . . The medical establishment may wink at false claims, but the insurance industry is less amused: it says about . . . $100 billion was lost to fraud [in 1999]."[52]

Health insurance carriers retaliate by "downcoding." Medicare carriers, complained psychiatrists, "are downcoding their claims for psychopharmacology services from 90862 to M0064—a code that is reimbursed at one-half the rate of 90862." (Code 90862 is for "Pharmacologic Management including prescription use," and Code M0064 for "Brief Office visit for the sole purpose of monitoring or changing drug prescriptions."[53]) The term "psychopharmacology services" is medical jargon for the psychiatrist's writing a prescription for a patient who wants or is willing to take a drug for what he thinks is a "chemical imbalance in his brain." Chester W. Schmidt, Jr., a psychiatrist at Johns Hopkins University Medical School and chairman of the American Psychiatric Association's (APA's) Work Group on Codes and Reimbursements, acknowledges that psychiatrists using "pharmacological management" do not physically examine their patients. Hence, they cannot possibly know what, if anything, is wrong with their brains.[54]

By the time the new century had arrived, the practice of making utterly false diagnoses of patients had become so frequent that it is now considered not just common but praiseworthy: it ennobles the physician as the compassionate savior of his patients, protecting them from greedy insurance companies. The following case is illustrative. On January 25, 2000, the *New York Times* reported that the federal government has filed an indictment for fraud against a prominent Manhattan gynecologist. "Prosecutors acknowledge that unlike doctors in most medical fraud cases, who bill for procedures that never took place or for patients who did not exist, Dr. X treated real patients for real conditions, treatments they were desperately seeking."[55] The problem was that the reimbursements for the procedures performed were excluded by the terms of the patients' health insurance policies. The case, commented the *Times,* "illuminates the quiet but common practice by doctors in many areas of medicine who tweak their bills to get approval or payment for treatments they believe patients need but insurance companies do not reimburse. A recent study in the *Archives of Internal Medicine* showed that 57 percent of 169 doctors who were polled said they would use deception to secure approval for certain treatments." In this particular case, Dr. X billed insurers for removing cysts and treating fibroids when, in fact, he was doing in vitro fertilizations. "According to the indictment, Dr. X told patients to lie about their care to investigators."

What is Dr X's defense? "It is ridiculous," he said, "that insurance companies will pay for a man to have Viagra but refuse to pay for a woman to have fertility treatments. I am completely innocent. I have never committed insurance fraud."[56] The doctor's lawyer argued "that what he [the doctor] did was treat 'real sick people.' . . . His defenders deny he committed fraud, or say it would have been justified if he did."[57] In documents submitted to the judge, the defense wrote: "The insurance companies allegedly victimized by this scheme were unlawfully discriminating against Dr. X's female patients by refusing to provide coverage for a 'disability' affecting a 'major life activity—reproduction.' In so doing, these insurance companies violated fundamental civil rights protected by the disabilities act." The best defense is an offense. A law professor comments: "It is still fraud. But there is a good chance that the jury will respond positively when they see real people up there."[58]

In Nazi Germany, the entire medical profession was corrupted, systematically lying to justify the euthanasia program. In the United States today, the entire medical profession is corrupted, systematically lying to justify a variety of medical interventions—especially for sexual and "mental" problems and the need for pain relief. A survey of physicians conducted by the AMA's Institute for Ethics revealed "strong support for the use of deception as a tool in six hypothetical situations," among them "pain medication for terminally ill patients" and "to secure third-party approval for patient procedures."[59]

It is no accident that the situations in which physicians feel most justified to lie concern the need and request for pain medication. Ironically, their incentive to lie in this situation is stimulated by the very drugs laws they enthusiastically support.[60] Doctors bitterly oppose the repeal of drug laws: Then, finding themselves constrained by them, they declare that it is "ethical" to evade them, "for the patient": "Sulmasy the ethicist is uncomfortable. . . . Sulmasy the physician is resolute: 'I feel I am doing something that is right and good on behalf of patients.' "[61] This rationalization can cover all bases.

Like many government programs, the DRGs began as a *permissive* system, permitting doctors to bill according to a schedule of diagnoses. The system is now de facto *prescriptive*, turning into diagnosis-related treatments (DRTs). (Diagnoses and treatments must "fit" together, like pieces of a puzzle.) Psychiatry again leads the parade. In 1999, United Health Care, the designated Medicare carrier for Connecticut, issued a set of draft regulations to providers of outpatient services covered under Medicare Part B: The regulations "would mandate that the treating physician prescribe medication to any patient diagnosed with one of the specified disorders, which include major depressive disorders, bipolar disorder, schizophrenic disorders, paranoid states, agoraphobia with or without panic attacks, social phobia, and obsessive-compulsive disorders. Failure to follow the protocol would result in nonreimbursement by Medicare."[62]

It is comforting, though, that all of these dreaded diseases can now be easily treated with pills.

DIAGNOSIS: THE CURRENCY OF THE THERAPEUTIC STATE

In the capitalist state, medical services are *exchanged* for money. In the therapeutic state, medical services are *provided* for diagnoses. To appreciate the significance of replacing money as a medium of exchange with diagnosis as a medium of justification, we must briefly consider the nature and function of money.

What Counts as Money?

Webster's International Dictionary devotes the better part of two pages to the various meanings of the word "money" and offers the following as its root meaning: "Something generally accepted as a medium of exchange, a measure of value, or a means of payment." In the *Oxford English Dictionary* (*OED*), with definitions of money running to more than five half-columns, the primary meaning of the word is given as: "Current coin; metal stamped in pieces of portable form as a medium of exchange and measure of value."

The difficulty of defining money descriptively led economists to suggest a functional definition for it. "Money," said the British economist Sir Ralph Hawley, "is one of those concepts . . . definable primarily by the use or purpose which they serve."[63] In other words, money, regardless of its physical or legal characteristics, may be anything that *functions as a device for exchanging and measuring wealth.* The point is that money is neither a production good, like machinery, nor a consumption good, like food; instead, it is a medium for *expressing a relationship among various goods.*

Almost any object that people value, especially if it is in short supply, can serve as a medium of exchange. In ancient times, commodities such as salt, sugar, tobacco, oxen, and slaves were so used. In Europe during and right after World War II, cigarettes were bartered for food and other necessities. The prohibition of certain commodities—today, so-called illegal drugs—often transforms them into forms of (illegal) currency, with profound social consequences.

From early times, ornamental, nonconsumable commodities, typically gold and silver, rather than useful, consumable objects, served as mediums of exchange. Through most of history, money was coinage, consisting of gold, silver, or some base metal, such as copper or nickel. Although the earliest use of paper money goes back to the second century B.C. in China, its entrance into the modern West is usually credited to, or blamed on, John Law, a colorful Scotsman perhaps best known as the architect of the infamous eighteenth-century speculative frenzy, the Mississippi (or Louisiana) Bubble.[64] However, not until the nineteenth century did paper money come into general use.

Economists distinguish among currency (or hand-to-hand circulating media, which includes coins and bank notes), money equivalents (such as demand bank deposits and treasury notes), and commodities used as money (such as gold or silver bullion or consumables such as tobacco). In modern industrial societies, coins and paper money form only a small part of a nation's total money supply, money equivalents accounting for the larger portion of it.

One of the characteristics of money is its connection to authority, hinted at in the etymology of the term. The word comes from the Latin "Moneta," as in the name of the Roman goddess Juno Moneta, in whose temple on the Capitoline Hill coin was minted and kept. In Latin, *monere* means to teach or instruct and *monitus,* a warning or admonition. The authority that legitimizes X as money may be a deity, a sovereign, a government, a bank, or a group of people. In fact, one of the principal characteristics of money may be said to lie in its being *accepted as currency*, a feature recognized by economists. To explain why money has value, they tell us, "it is necessary to introduce acceptability; i.e., behavior."[65] The same goes for diagnosis: a word functions as a diagnosis only if it is accepted as the name of a disease. Accordingly, a person with a diagnosis is generally accepted as ill and deserving of treatment, while a person without a diagnosis is generally viewed as not ill and hence not deserving of medical attention. These aspects of the term "diagnosis" underscore its important functions as a *medium of exchange*—between everyman *qua* patient and everyone else with whom he interacts (family, physicians, nurses, employers, insurance companies, lawyers, the state), and among the diverse individuals and institutions that interact with one another in matters relating to persons-qua-patients (physicians and pharmacists, physicians and state medical licensing authorities, pharmacists and the Drug Enforcement Agency [DEA], and so forth).

Standards: Monetary and Medical

The medium of exchange used as money is called the "monetary standard." Such standards are of two types, commodity standards (precious metal) and noncommodity standards (paper, or so-called "fiat money"). The term "fiat money" comes from the Latin *fiat* for "let there be," as in *Fiat lux ("Let* there be light!") in the Latin bible. Fiat money is paper transformed into money by the decree of the state.

The term "gold standard" refers to fixing the value of a unit of currency by pegging it to a stipulated amount (weight) of gold. From the Middle Ages until World War I, currencies based on gold, usually gold coins, were the norm. Nonmetallic money was little used in Europe before the end of the eighteenth century. In the United States, gold coins and gold certificates ceased to function as legal tender in 1934. Since the middle 1930s, virtually all governments have adopted the fiat standard for their money, freeing them from any obligation to repay the holders of coins or bank notes in gold or silver. The volume of currency the world over, including American currency, is now limited only by the actions of governments, and not by the supply of precious metals (whose availability is not under the direct control of the state).

Although privately issued money has existed from time to time—and privately issued money equivalents abound (bonds, stocks, etc.)—most people assume that issuing money *must be* a state monopoly. This perception is embedded in our language, the medium of exchange officially designated as money being called "legal tender," which *Webster's* defines as: "that currency, or money, which the law authorizes a debtor to tender and requires a creditor to receive in payment of money obligations." It is this idea that allows for the transformation of an intrinsically worthless commodity (paper) into a fiscally valuable entity (fiat money as legal tender), and makes monetary inflation (and deflation) possible.

As standards of money have ranged from salt and slaves to gold and silver, so standards of disease (and hence disease names) have ranged from humoral imbalances to bodily lesions. During the better part of the barely 200-year history of scientific medicine, its standard of illness has been somatic pathology.[66] Like the gold standard of money, the *somatic-pathological standard pegs diagnosis to an objectively fixed criterion of disease*—a "thing" that cannot be created capriciously or at the command of the government. In sum:

- The gold monetary standard makes the creation of *new* legal tender contingent on the acquisition (production) of new stores of gold. The government can create more money only by having miners mine more gold. The fiat monetary standard allows the government to create money simply by having printers print more of it.

- The gold disease standard makes the creation of *new* medical diagnoses contingent on the *discovery of new scientifically defined diseases.* Physicians and the government can create more diseases only by having scientists discover more diseases. The fiat medical standard allows physicians and the government to create more diseases simply by having doctors create more diagnoses.

The analogy is instructive. Under the gold standard, creditors do not have to accept payments in materials other than gold (or moneys backed by gold). Similarly, under the gold medical standard, critics of medical imperialism do not have to accept diagnoses unless they are backed by objective pathological findings of disease.

However, each system has an escape clause, a crucial exception: any crisis credibly labeled an "emergency" legitimizes abandoning the standard. In wartimes, "national emergency" justified governments on the gold standard to issue fiat money. In much the same way, war plus compulsory military service led physicians to abandon the scientific standard of disease and issue fiat diagnoses. Thus arose the concept of "trauma" as a cause of disease. In World War I, malingering was called "shell shock," as if it were a neurological disease, or "soldier's heart," as if it were a cardiac disease. In World War II, it was called "battle fatigue," "combat fatigue," or was legitimized as a "neurosis," typically "traumatic neurosis." These conditions, Jonas Robitscher cogently observed, "had achieved legitimacy as diseases."[67] The "patients" were called "neuropsychiatric casualties" and typically were discharged and awarded disability compensation for suffering from a "neuropsychiatric disorder." The war against mental illness—together with the wars against drugs, gambling, smoking, and other disapproved behaviors—has produced a diagnostic inflation comparable to the monetary inflation of post–World War I Germany. During World Wars I and II, most people preferred to deny that men were excused and discharged from the service because they were afraid of being injured, killed, or simply did not want to serve. Similarly, in our day of metaphorical world wars, most people prefer to believe that gambling, smoking, illicit drug use, and mental illnesses are real diseases.

It is important to keep in mind that, from ancient times until the nineteenth century, there was no firm linkage between disease and lesion: *virtually all diagnoses then were fiat diagnoses.* (Terms such as "dropsy" and "gout" and some others are exceptions to this rule.) Decisive advances in medical epistemology and medical ethics occurred partly as the result of the creation of the gold standard of disease qua somatic lesion.

The first modern psychiatric fiat diseases were manic-depression and dementia praecox, attributed to and perceived as brain diseases. By 1911, when Bleuler renamed dementia praecox "schizophrenia," it was uncontested medical dogma that insane persons suffered from incurable brain diseases and presented a permanent danger to the public, justifying their incarceration in insane asylums. The idea that mental patients are hospitalized for their own welfare and treatment is a post–World War II flourish. The fact that, from its earliest origins, psychiatry was a purely statist enterprise is consistent with and strongly supports this interpretation. The functions the state assigned to psychiatrists were similar to those it assigned to prison guards, rather than to those it assigned to privately practicing physicians.

As the gold monetary standard obligates the government to redeem paper money in gold, so the gold medical standard obligates the medical profession to grant disease status to diagnoses only if they can be "redeemed" by demonstrating that they name somatic pathology. This is more than an analogy. The notion of redeeming diagnosis for disease continues to play a crucial role in medicine (as contrasted with psychiatry). In the academic-medical exercise known as the "clinical-pathological conference," an audience of physicians and medical students is presented with the "case" of a sick person, the clinical diagnosis made by his attending physician, and the pathological diagnosis made by the pathologist at autopsy (or by biopsy). To the extent that the clinical diagnosis fails to match the pathological diagnosis, the practicing physician's diagnosis is deemed to be erroneous. The fact that a clinical-pathological conference on the case of a patient with mental illness is an oxymoron is *prima facie* evidence that psychiatric diagnoses do not name "diseases" with somatic markers and hence are, by definition, not diseases.

The fiat monetary standard grants the government the authority and power to treat paper money as legal tender, letting the quantity of legal tender increase independently of any increase in gold backing its value. Similarly, the fiat diagnostic standard grants the medical profession and the government the authority and power to treat words that sound like the names of diseases as if they were diseases, or to use "real disease" terminology for nondiseases, letting medically and legally legitimated diagnoses increase independently of any evidence of somatic pathology backing their disease status. This is why psychiatric nosology is highly unstable; why, especially since the end of Wold War II, there has been a veritable explosion in the diagnoses of new mental diseases; and why the rosters of mental disorders are regularly revised, old diagnoses (such as homosexuality) being delisted, and new diagnoses (such as attention deficit hyperactivity disorder) being added.

Inflation: Undermining the Integrity of Symbols

Orderly human relations depends on the proper functioning of speech, speakers and listeners attaching *the same meaning* to words. The languages we speak and how well or poorly we speak them define who we are and largely determine who the persons near and dear to us are. Words have standardized meanings: Dictionaries are the telephone directories of languages. Safeguarding the fixity of the meaning of words (and other symbols) is essential for the integrity and pursuit of the sciences and is indispensable for law, economics, commerce, and honest dealing among upright persons. Conversely, corrupting the meaning of words undermines their integrity, obstructs cultural and scientific progress, and hinders honest discourse among people.

Anchoring money in an objective standard (gold) serves the interests of free trade, the security of property, and personal liberty. Anchoring diagnosis in an objective standard (somatic pathology) serves the interests of medical science, sound medical practice, and personal liberty. Dislodging the meaning of these symbols from their precisely defined positions—legitimizing fiat money and fiat diagnosis as "real" money and real diagnosis—serves the interests of the new political class, the pharmacrats.

As long as the gold standard was the accepted measure of money, no abstract monetary standard, or "numeraire," was needed; similarly, as long as the gold standard of disease was the accepted measure of disease, no abstract disease standard, or "diagnostic numeraire," was needed.[68] The term "numeraire" is recent coinage. The *Supplement to the Oxford English Dictionary* defines it as "the function of money as a measure of value or unit of account," and dates its origin to 1964. When nations relinquish the gold standard, the English pound, American dollar, or the euro becomes the numeraire. When medicine relinquishes the gold standard of disease, *the profession's diagnostic manuals be-*

come the medical numeraire. This is the background against which we must view the current diagnostic inflation.

We have fixed standards for time, length, weight, and so forth, and do not debate how many minutes there are in an hour or how many inches in a yard. If we ask, Why don't we have a fixed standard for disease?, the answer is, we do, but we no longer adhere to it. For example, although Aronowitz recognizes the prevailing diagnostic inflation and writes "that we might question whether we need to cap or develop some standards for legitimating the explosion of these *ill*ness-less' diagnoses,"[69] he fails to mention the pathological standard for legitimating disease or the name of Rudolf Virchow.

Emperors, dictators, and democratic governments alike finance wars by creating excess money, that is, by monetary inflation. Similarly, therapeutic states finance their wars on mental illnesses, drugs, and other bad habits or unwanted behaviors by diagnostic inflation. During the past twenty years, numerous authors and publications, in professional journals and the popular press alike, have criticized and ridiculed one or another aspect of the medicalization of life—without, however, telling us what they regard as the objective standard of disease.[70]

The term "medicalization" is part of the problem: it implies that something is being treated as if it were a medical problem when, "in fact," it is not a medical problem. Consider, in this connection, the analogous phenomenon of the "theologization of life": the term implies that something is being treated as if it were a religious problem when, in fact, it is not a religious problem. However, for people obsessed with worshiping God, everything is a religious matter. Similarly, for people obsessed with worshiping health, everything is a medical matter.

CONCLUSIONS

Nosology, or the classification of disease, depends on what counts as a disease. Classic nosology was *descriptive,* based on *pathology.* Contemporary nosology is *strategic,* based on *economic, legal, social, and other interests, unrelated to disease as somatic pathology.* The clinician as middleman between the patient and the health care bureaucracy makes diagnoses to legitimize treatment, to secure reimbursement for medical services, to justify defining undesirable behavior as disease, and so forth. DRGs provide medical-economic rationale for fixing the value/cost of medical services reimbursed by third-party payers. Psychiatric diagnoses provide medical-legal rationale for treating mental diseases as if they were brain diseases, excusing guilty persons of crimes, confining innocent persons as dangerous, and so forth.

Formerly, diagnoses encoded the objectively verifiable, somatic-pathological condition of the patient's body, that is, diseases. Today, diagnoses rationalize the health-care policy of the body politic, that is, they determine physician compensation, control medical costs, justify patient coercion, and so forth. During the past half century, we have witnessed the transformation of nosology from the medical-scientific classification of disease as somatic pathology to the medicalized rationalization of government regulation as "health care."

4

CERTIFYING MEDICINE
Disability

Nothing is so difficult to distinguish as the nuances which separate un-merited misfortune from an adversity produced by vice.

Alexis de Tocqueville[1]

Most of the world's work is done by people who don't feel very well.

Winston Churchill[2]

The conventional image of medicine, consisting of the physician as medical scientist or medical practitioner, is incomplete. Missing is a familiar aspect of medicine that has no name. I suggest we call it "certifying medicine," because it is characterized by the primary or sole role of the physician, or other health-care professional, being that of a certifying agent. The certifying physician may function as an agent of an individual or as an agent of an institution or the state. Psychiatry rests on the denial of this elementary fact. Herein, also, lies one of the unrecognized dangers of third-party payments for medical care and, more generally, of all systems of socialized health care.

Typically, the certifying physician functions as an agent of the party that seeks his help and pays for his services. For example, he helps a person secure a prescription drug, deferment from military service, relief from jury duty, or a handicapped parking permit. Or he helps an institution, whose interests may differ or oppose those of the patient, for example, to solve a crime, as a coroner; declare a soldier fit or unfit for duty, as a military physician; prevent a person with an infectious disease from working as a food handler, as a public health physician.

The more socially and technologically complex society becomes, the more the role of the physician as certifying agent expands. In the United States today, the role of the physician as certifying agent is perhaps even greater and more important than is his role as healer. In this chapter, I consider one of the physician's paradigmatic certifying roles, defining and determining what counts as disability. In the next chapter, I consider another, closely related medical-certifying role, namely, defining and determining what counts as mental illness.

THE PROBLEM OF DISABILITY

For animals in the wild, disability—a "condition that incapacitates in any way" (*Webster's*)—is tantamount to a death sentence. The only exceptions may be the very young of some species, protected by their mothers, or sometimes fathers. In contrast, animals cared for and useful to man—creatures in zoos, household pets, farm animals—can and often do survive in an incapacitated state. In fact, Americans now seem more willing to spend *their own money* on veterinary care for their pets than on medical care for themselves. A distinguishing feature of a civilized society is its willingness to aid and protect its disabled members and refrain from needlessly destroying animals and plants.

Historically, disability has been an enormous problem for human beings, not only for the individuals affected but also for those dependent on them. The paradigmatic disability is infancy, and the paradigmatic institution for its mitigation is the family, especially the mother, her protective function epitomized by feeding the young with a product of her own body. The oldest social agency for the relief of disability is the church. The participation of the state in the determination and palliation of disability is a recent development.

Defining Disability

Webster's defines disability as "deprivation or lack, esp. of physical, intellectual, or emotional capacity or fitness; a physical or mental illness, injury, or condition that incapacitates in any way. . . . the inability to pursue an occupation or perform services for wages because of physical or mental impairment; handicap; lack of legal qualification (incompetence); disadvantage." Note that disability is here defined as a condition (noun), not as an attribute (adjective). More succinctly, The *Oxford English Dictionary* (*OED*) defines disability as "want of ability (to discharge any office or function); inability, incapacity, impotence."

Henry H. Kessler, M.D., widely acknowledged as the father of modern American disability evaluations, states: "The term 'disability' denotes a physical defect or impairment and the resulting social and economic status of the affected individual. . . . medical assessment plays a dominant, and often the only, role in the final judicial decision concerning disability claims. . . . *Gross error occurs only when the standards of evaluation are insufficiently grounded in anatomical and physiological reality.*"[3] This claim is patently erroneous: It may be false, as when disability is attributed to nondisabling physical illness; and it is always and necessarily false when it is attributed to mental illness, which cannot be diagnosed by physical signs or laboratory findings.

The U.S. Department of Commerce is charged with keeping statistics about the incidence of disability in the population. According to this agency, "a person is considered to *have a disability* if he or she has difficulty performing certain functions (seeing, hearing, walking, climbing stairs and lifting and carrying) . . . or has difficulty with certain social roles (doing school work for children, working at a job and around the house for adults)."[4] "Severe disability" is defined as a condition "requiring the use of an assistive device or assistance from another person to perform basic activities," a criterion that places anyone who needs reading glasses, hearing aids, dentures, or protective clothing or even sunscreen in the class of the "severely disabled." Not surprisingly, 1 in 5 Americans is said to have "some kind of disability" and 1 in 10 to have "a severe disability."[5]

There are important similarities between conflating disease and disability and conflating bodily disease and mental disease. Like mental illness, disability is a highly elastic term and category. Indeed, according to the Supreme Court, "no agency has been delegated authority to interpret the term 'disability.' "[6] As a result, the term includes many voluntary (mis)behaviors—for example, alcoholism—validated as medical disabilities by the Americans with Disabilities Act of 1990 (AWDA). What began as the manufacture of madness in the eighteenth century became the manufacture of disability in the twentieth century.[7]

According to the Department of Commerce, a major purpose of the AWDA "was to increase the employment rate of people with disabilities by making it illegal to practice discrimination against individuals who *happen to have a disability.*"[8] The Act was promoted for and by people with physical problems who *wanted to work,* but whom others viewed as too disabled to do so. Being disabled, we must keep in mind, a social role that a person *seeks or avoids,* as the case may be. Furthermore, disability may be the result of a self-inflicted injury or illness, for example, cirrhosis from drinking, lung cancer from smoking. The currently accepted, expansive definitions of disability rest not only on a denial of the ability to function in general despite major handicaps, but also on a denial of the ubiquity of malingering and the true nature of so-called mental illnesses.[9]

Being disabled, like being sick, is a *role* that is assumed or claimed by a person, or is ascribed to and imposed on him. In the case of bodily illness, people assume the disabled role voluntarily, to obtain money or goods or services that cannot be purchased in the marketplace, such as prescription drugs, special parking permits, or military deferments. In the case of mental illness, people sometimes assume the disabled role willingly, indeed eagerly, to obtain room and board in a mental hospital or receive compensation; sometimes the role is imposed on them against their will: on law-abiding persons in order to deprive them of liberty by civil commitment, and on lawbreakers in order to deprive them of their constitutional right to trial by declaring them mentally unfit. One of the tragicomic consequences of our mental illness and disability practices is the ex-mental patient who stoutly denies the reality of mental illness, but feels entitled to collect disability benefits for it.

Determining Disability: Disease or Social Role?

Formerly, able-bodied beggars faked being crippled and wealthy debtors pretended to be destitute.[10] Today, hundreds of thousands of people able to work claim to be disabled, physically or mentally, to avoid supporting themselves. As the history of poor relief is largely the record of efforts to separate the "deserving" from the "undeserving" poor,[11] so the history of disability compensation is largely the record of efforts to separate persons who deserve disability benefits from those who do not.

It is self-evident that disability—"impairment," in the official jargon—may or may not be the result of disease. Nevertheless, the Advisory Council to the Social Security Board mandates "that compensable disabilities be restricted to those which can be *objectively determined by medical examination or tests.* . . . Unless demonstrable by objective tests, such ailments as lumbago, rheumatism, and various nervous disorders would not be compensable. The danger of malingering which might be involved in connection with such claims would thereby be avoided."[12] Ironically, *DSM-IV* defines malingering as a bona fide mental disorder, also called factitious disorder or Munchausen syndrome. (Psychiatrists do not classify feigning health by denying illness as factitious health and the condition does not qualify the sufferer for disability status.)

A 1967 amendment to the regulations of the Social Security Act restated: "For purposes of this subsection, 'a physical or mental impairment' is an impairment *that results from anatomical, physiological, or psychological abnormalities which are demonstrable by medically acceptable clinical and laboratory diagnostic techniques.*"[13] In 1976, this "fictitious truth"—plainly inconsistent with the actual practices used to determine disability—received the imprimatur of the Supreme Court, which held that, to discontinue disability benefits, "a medical assessment of the worker's physical or mental condition is required. . . . the decision whether to discontinue disability benefits will turn, in most cases, upon routine, standard, and *unbiased medical reports by physician specialists.*"[14] This concept of disability illustrates what may be called a "definitional belief," similar to the belief that human beings officially classified as "slaves" are property, or that prisons called "mental hospitals" are hospitals.

Unfortunately, it is often difficult to distinguish genuine disability from deliberate deception. Formerly, physicians and even medical organizations acknowledged this limitation of the medical role. In 1956, a representative of the American Academy of General Practice protested: "Medical science has not reached the point of being able to unerringly state whether or not a man is totally and permanently disabled. . . . Is the delivery boy who loses both legs totally and permanently disabled? Or is the certifying doctor supposed to point out that he can still run a drill press and probably make more money?"[15] Regardless of how far medical science may advance, a certifying doctor will never be "able to unerringly state whether or not a man is totally and permanently disabled." However, the bureaucracy needed experts to separate the disabled from the nondisabled and declared that doctors can do the job. "No matter what physicians said"—concludes Deborah A. Stone, professor of political science at the Massachusetts Institute of Technology—"nothing could shake Congressional belief in the ability of the medical profession to make reasonably accurate judgments of disability."[16] This remains the case today, reinforced by the American Medical Association's official *Guides to the Evaluation of Permanent Impairment.*[17]

Notwithstanding the tenuous link between disease and disability, the gatekeeper posted at the entrance to the role of disabled person is the physician. The claims process *must begin* with a physician examining the claimant and giving him a *diagnosis.* No diagnosis, no disability. Stone correctly emphasizes that "medical certification of disability has become one of the major paths to public aid in the modern welfare state."[18] More importantly for our present purposes, this policy is a bottomless source of fictitious diseases, that is, diagnoses required as evidence of the putative *causes* of the subject's disability. "One can only marvel or despair," Stone continues, "at the technicalization of a political issue, when the technical experts themselves insist on the inability of their science to perform the tasks expected of it."[19] Why shouldn't politicians believe that physicians can make scientifically reliable disability determinations if physicians are willing to do precisely that?

Our disability and welfare policies promote not only malingering and filing false claims for disability, but also self-indulgent self-neglect, such as drug abuse.

In a study covering 165,000 random deaths, investigators found that "the number of deaths is higher in the first week of the month than in the last week of the preceding month."[20] This cycle parallels the cycle of payments for needs-based benefits: "Payments for many types of federal benefits, such as Social Security, welfare, and military benefits, typically arrive at the beginning of each month. . . . Money for purchasing drugs or alcohol tends to be available at the beginning of the month and is relatively less available (for people with low incomes) at the end of the month when discretionary funds maybe exhausted."[21] This hypothesis is supported by the fact that the excessive deaths at the beginning of each month are due largely to drug abuse, homicide, suicide, and accident.

The medicalization of disability represents a giant step in the transformation of the welfare state into the therapeutic state. While the two systems resemble one another, both being need-based and paternalistic, there are important differences between them:

- The welfare state seeks to *relieve poverty and unemployment;* its beneficiaries are not helped against their will; it is a constitutional state, regulated by the rule of law.
- The therapeutic state seeks to *remedy personal and social problems defined as diseases;* its beneficiaries are often helped against their will; it is a totalitarian state, governed by the rule of therapeutic discretion.

DISABILITY: PATIENT VERSUS SOCIETY

Although illness and injury often result in disability, disability is *not* synonymous with disease and is *not* a purely medical concept; it is a *judgment about an individual's ability to perform a particular task*. Everyone may be said to be "disabled" *relative* to his own maximum ability, to certain tasks, or to the abilities of more competent others. A short person is disabled from being a professional basketball player, a heavy person from being a jockey, an illiterate person from virtually all work in an advanced society. None, however, has a disease. A sick person may or may not be disabled or may be disabled for a shorter or longer period (from earning a living). Whether a person is disabled from being gainfully employed or working as an independent producer depends less on his medical condition than on his educational level, motivation for work, and the personal, economic, and political opportunities open to him. Nevertheless, the concepts of disease and disability are typically yoked together, with medical certification for disability focused on what the subject *cannot* do because of his *medical impairment*, rather than on what he *can do in spite of it*.

Want, Need, and Disability

Although disease may cause disability, the connection between disease and disability is rarely a matter of direct cause and effect. Sick persons may be unable to do physical labor but be able to do other useful work. Conversely, healthy persons, able to work, may claim to be disabled and may be so classified. Persons may *falsely claim* or *falsely disclaim* being disabled.

The fallacy of inferring disability from disease is dramatically illustrated by the different attitudes of VIPs and VUPs toward *claiming and disclaiming the disabled role.* The typical VIP has a prestigious position, clings to his job and the status it gives him, and denies or minimizes the disabilities imposed on him by disease or aging. Franklin Roosevelt was paralyzed by polio. Dwight Eisenhower suffered from chronic colitis and had a heart attack while in office. John Kennedy suffered from Addison's disease and complications from its treatment with steroids. None of these VIPs wanted to be viewed or treated as disabled. Stephen Hawking, severely disabled by amyotrophic lateral sclerosis, is a professor at Cambridge University and a best-selling author with an annual income in excess of a million pounds (about 1.6 million dollars).[22]

Conversely, the typical VUP is unemployed or has a menial job with low status that he may be eager to exchange for the more respectable and lucrative role of a victim disabled by disease. In addition to enhancing his status, such an exchange may *exempt* him from certain obligations and may *entitle* him to certain benefits, for example, housing, food, money, perhaps even fame. Indeed, being viewed as disabled may enhance a person's social status and may result in his receiving more money and services than he could have earned if he had not been disabled. Before his attempt to assassinate President Ronald Reagan, John W. Hinckley, Jr. was an aimless college dropout, shunned by his family. In 1982, he committed his (in)famous deed and was declared not responsible for it by reason of mental illness. Now he plays the role of a famous madman disabled by a dreadful disease. "At one time," he boasts, "Miss [Jody] Foster was a star and I was the insignificant fan. Now everything is changed. I am Napoleon and she is Josephine. I am Romeo and she is Juliet. . . . I'm famous as hell."[23]

What makes a person like Hinckley *disabled?* His *ability* to shoot others, a premeditated crime that *we interpret* as a *disability due to a disease.* Disability produced by deviant ability is as different from disability due to physical limitation as mental illness is different from bodily illness. The "bizarre act" of a so-called mental patient, whether murder or self-mutilation, is a complex performance, an ability most people lack. In contrast, the disability of a physically sick person, such as blindness or paralysis, is the absence of an innate sensory or motor ability, not the lack of a social skill or the rejection of responsibility. Attributing adult dependency to disabling disease is as fallacious and misguided as is attributing crime to mental illness.

James D. Davidson and William Rees-Mogg cogently observe: "An increase in the repertoire of skills required to earn income in the market automatically increases the relative attractiveness of seeking what one wants by violence.

Crime is easier than calculus."[24] Malingering is easier than digging ditches. Nevertheless, in the therapeutic state, politicians, physicians, and the public tend to accept and are encouraged to accept that unwillingness or inability to support oneself is a disease or is due to a disease. Rejecting this belief is politically incorrect. The intimate connection between insanity and disability is supported by the centuries-old legal and social recognition of mental illness as *a disabling condition for which the subject is not responsible.* Such a connection is intrinsic to the discipline of psychiatry as a branch of medical science and medical practice. The chronic mental patient may thus be a double "beneficiary": he is paid for his illness *and* is deemed not guilty of a crime when he pushes someone under the subway.

Like the undefinable concept of mental illness, the undefinable concept of medical disability is widely accepted because it is socially useful, indeed indispensable: Both constructs enable society to treat *existential-vocational problems as diseases,* justifying the special legal status of the subjects as victims, and authorizing monetary payment to them; both advance the basic goal of the therapeutic state—to replace a want-based with a need-based system of distributing goods and services.

Disability as a Social-Economic and Political Problem

The problem of disability, as we know it, did not exist before the advent of modernity.[25] In ancient Greece and Rome, soldiers disabled in war received a pension from the state. That arrangement, however, was an isolated *quid pro quo.* When the state needed the free citizen to defend the nation, he came to its aid. When the veteran became old and destitute, the state reciprocated. The principle that it is the *obligation of the state* to provide relief to workers disabled by their occupation—or to any disabled person—is a late nineteenth-century notion, developed in Germany and then adopted by other nations.

In the United States today, millions of people receive disability benefits from numerous agencies and programs, such as Social Security Disability Insurance, Social Security Supplemental Security Income, Medicare, Medicaid, Workman's Compensation, and private health and disability insurance companies. Since the 1960s, when the Social Security Disability Insurance program became part of the Social Security System, virtually everyone considered "disabled from gainful employment," regardless of age or employment record, has become eligible to receive payment for disability.

Like the welfare system, the disability system is need-based. The authorities in charge of the system must separate *truly needy persons not responsible for their plight* from *persons who pretend to be needy or are responsible for their plight.* To protect itself from abuses, the disability system creates a bureaucracy to limit entry into the system: Its primary gatekeeper, as we saw, is the physician, with administrators, judges, and courts serving as the final arbiters. Despite all efforts, it is impossible to prevent the system from being overused and thus abused. This system failure is intrinsic to all need-based mechanisms for distributing goods or services.

- In a want-based system, A pays B for the goods or services he wants, and B receives the money he needs. We call this capitalism and the market.

- In a need-based system, if A wants certain goods or services from B, he must request C to authorize B to deliver them. Both B and C are paid by the state (taxpayer). We call this socialism and guaranteeing "social justice."

In the need-based system, even if A's need is genuine, he must *claim* it; that is, he must communicate it to the proper authorities in appropriate ways. To be successful, A may also have to exaggerate his need. Finally, if A's need is not genuine—if he wants certain goods or services not because he needs them but, say, because he wants to avoid some obligation—then he must fake his need. Hence the waggish observation that there are only two economic systems, capitalism and corruption.

It is no secret that distinguishing needy persons from fakers can be very difficult in practice. Testifying before a Congressional committee, a Social Security Commissioner stated: "The phrase 'by reason of any medically determinable physical or mental impairment' is part of the definition [of disability] that administratively gives us the most trouble and yet is really absolutely essential to the definition."[26] Replace the phrase "by reason of any medically determinable physical or mental impairment," with the phrase "by reason of any medically determinable insanity," and we find the classic McNaghten Rule, the familiar legal-psychiatric formula for transforming murderers destined for execution into mental patients not responsible for their criminal acts. The formula is worthless because it masks a strategic economic, criminologic, political decision as a descriptive medical, technical determination.

Transforming disability from an existential disaster into an economic bonanza has, of course, far-reaching financial, personal, political, and social consequences. Long before the advent of Medicare, Medicaid, and the AWDA, Ludwig von Mises warned: "As a social institution it [social insurance] has thus made the neurosis of the insured a dangerous public disease. Should the institution be extended and developed the disease will spread. . . . We cannot weaken or destroy the will to health without producing illness."[27]

It is widely recognized that once a disability program is established, its cost becomes politically uncontrollable, partly because the very existence of the program becomes an incentive for the production of more disability.[28] Although in advanced societies certain kinds of disability policies may be necessary, the problems they inevitably create ought not to be minimized or medicalized. In particular, we must be vigilant about the ways in which our ideas about disability contaminate and confuse our ideas about disease, and vice versa.

Disability: Involuntary Condition or Voluntary Strategy?

The term "disability" may name an involuntary condition, the unwanted result of an injury or illness, or a voluntary strategy, the effort to obtain benefits by nonmonetary means. It is difficult to distinguish between these phenomena, especially if, as is the case at present, doing so is widely viewed as politically incorrect. "Disability studies" are now an academic subject on college campuses: "Debates are now underway on whether able-bodied professors will be allowed to teach disabilities and whether contributions to the culture by the mentally disabled will be covered."[29] Such a development bodes ill for a dispassionate study of the subject.

Disfranchised or otherwise politically enfeebled individuals—children, slaves, prisoners, military personnel—are often compelled to perform duties that are, or seem to them, arduous, dangerous, unpleasant. They have few options for easing their burden. They can kill themselves. They can escape, if there is a place of refuge to which they can flee. Or they can pretend to be disabled, assuming the authorities regard disability as an excusing condition.[30] It would be futile for a child who does not want to go to school to tell his mother that he would prefer to stay home. However, if he fibs and tells her that he feels sick and fakes a fever by surreptitiously heating a thermometer, he is likely to accomplish his goal.

Novels, biographies, and autobiographies abound with accounts of malingering. In the *Confessions of Felix Krull,* Thomas Mann presents the hilarious tale of a young man's artfully orchestrated performance aimed at securing his rejection from military service during World War I.[31] A similar true story is told by James Gleick in *Genius*, a biography of the physicist Richard Feynman. Called up for the service, the examining psychiatrist asks Feynman if he ever "hears voices." Mockingly, Feynman says "yes," and, like Felix Krull, is declared mentally unfit for service.[32]

The recognition that some people are genuinely ill while others are "deserters from life" long antedates the development of modern medicine and the scientific concept of disease. In the *Republic*, Plato inveighs against the physician who accepts the malingerer as a *bona fide* patient and treats his complaints as if they were real diseases: "[T]o require medicine, said I, not merely for wounds or the incidence of some seasonal maladies, but, because of sloth and such a regimen as we described, to fill one's body up with winds and humors like a marsh and compel the ingenious sons of Asclepius *to invent for diseases such names as fluxes and flatulences*—don't you think that disgraceful?"[33]

Plato objected to the physician's validating laziness as an illness. The modern physician makes a medical virtue out of what Plato considered a medical vice. As practicing physician, he often diagnoses discomforts as diseases, to please the patient. As psychiatrist, he *imposes diagnoses of mental illnesses on persons against their will, to discredit their mental competence and obscure the true meaning of their behavior.*[34]

The proposition that it ought to be the duty of the state to provide compensation to workmen disabled by their labors was first made national policy by Chancellor Otto von Bismarck. It is now generally believed that Bismarck was concerned about the welfare of the workers. Nothing could be further from the truth. He was concerned about the well-being of the *German state*. In a message to the Reichstag, the Emperor, articulating Bismarck's aim, requested "legislation for the measure that will make possible the solution of the problems which prevent the *Sovereign Power from flourishing to the full on its own.*"[35] The first German "Sickness Insurance Law" was enacted in 1884.

Despite his passionate interest in preventive medicine, Rudolf Virchow, the foremost medical man of the day as well as a Reichstag deputy, opposed the measure.[36] He did so because he realized that its aim was political, not medical. Bismarck hated Communism. He introduced socialized medicine into Germany to buy the loyalty of the German masses: Bismarck "adopted 'nationalistic socialism to end international socialism.' . . . [He] was the first leader of a great nation to fight Communism by adopting Communism. . . . [His scheme] became an important feature of the German militaristic state; it helped pave the way for Hitler a generation later."[37] I would add that Bismarck's nationalization of medicine paved the way not only for Hitler but also, more specifically, for the Nazi program of medicalized mass murder, and, more generally, for the triumph of the therapeutic state and the prevailing political incorrectness of opposing it.[38]

The agency entrusted with administering the German sickness insurance was called the *Krankenkasse*, or sickness office. Fearing that free choice of physicians would lead to "overutilization as a result of malingering [and] would milk the funds dry," the administrators of the *Krankenkassen* opposed the patient's right to choose his own physician.[39] Inevitably, the system lent a powerful impetus to the human inclination to malinger. To combat abuses, the *Krankenkassen* soon created a special corps of physicians, called *"Vertrauensärzte"* (trusted physicians). Their job was to reexamine patients certified as disabled by officially authorized *Krankenkasse* doctors. In their well-documented book

Medicine and the State, Matthew J. Lynch and Stanley S. Raphael, two Canadian pathologists, report on a study of disabled employees of three Berlin companies ordered to be reexamined by *Vertrauensärzte:* "between 18.3 percent and 26.5 percent declared themselves fit immediately," that is without reexamination; about 25 percent to 30 percent of those remaining were found fit on reexamination. Before World War II, more than 50 percent of the workers certified as sick in Vienna were found to be "healthy enough for work." After the war, the old patten quickly reemerged. In a 1953 study conducted in Germany, out of some 85,000 claimants for sick pay ordered to be examined by trust physicians, more than half failed to present themselves for examination.[40]

In the Soviet Union, the physician was, *ipso facto*, the agent of the state. His primary role was "that of a *certifying agent*."[41]

Malingering, Mental Illness, and Disability

Mad-doctors have always insisted on three interlinked propositions, namely: that all of their patients are insane; that no sane person is ever confined in an insane asylum; and that insanity is a condition that befalls people against their will. When the mad-doctors metamorphosed into psychiatrists, they decided that it does not matter whether a crazy person *is* crazy or only *acts* crazy: in either case, he must be crazy and hence merits being classified as ill. The idea that pretending to be mentally ill is itself an illness is one of psychiatry's most inspired deceptions.

In 1924, Eugen Bleuler, the inventor of schizophrenia, declared: "Those who simulate insanity with some cleverness are nearly all psychopaths and some are actually insane. Demonstration of simulation, therefore, does not at all prove that the patient is mentally sound and responsible for his actions."[42] Ironically, the scientific-medical bankruptcy of the idea of mental illness became the foundation for the empire of modern psychiatry.

During World War II, the proposition that faking disease is, itself, a disabling illness became an integral part of "humane" military-medical practice. After the war, it became psychiatric dogma. Kurt Eissler, a world-famous psychoanalyst and psychiatrist, framed the doctrine thus: "It can be rightly claimed that malingering is *always the sign of a disease* . . . which to diagnose requires particularly keen diagnostic acumen. . . . It is a great mistake to make the patient suffering from the disease liable to prosecution."[43]

DSM-IV defines malingering, coded V65.2, as "the intentional production of false or grossly exaggerated physical or psychological symptoms, motivated by external incentives."[44] This is a pretentious circumlocution for feigning illness. Factitious disorders—coded 300.16 or 300.19 depending on whether "psychological or physical signs and symptoms" predominate—are defined as "characterized by physical or psychological symptoms that are intentionally produced or feigned in order to assume the sick role."[45] The APA thus validates a type of *conduct that it acknowledges to be a species of voluntary behavior* as a mental disorder. It compounds this folly by adding: "A Factitious Disorder must be distinguished from a true medical condition and from true mental disorder."[46] But if a true mental disorder is a *bona fide* true medical condition, why must a factitious disorder be distinguished from *both*?

The proposition that mental disorders are medical diseases (brain diseases) is a big lie. Big lies cannot be concealed forever, as the following examples illustrate.

On March 9, 1989, Anthony M. Rizzo, Jr., an administrator and teacher in the Fairfax, Virginia school system for twenty-five years, was fired by the school board after seven teachers and an administrator accused him of sexual harassment. Rizzo denied all the allegations. However, while Rizzo denied harassing the teachers throughout the dispute over his pension, "his lawyer was citing the harassment as evidence of Rizzo's disability." Robert S. Brown, Jr., Rizzo's psychiatrist, certified that his client was suffering from "a personality disorder with 'narcissistic' features and a psychosexual disorder," and explained that "if Rizzo were placed in any job where he was supervising women, his psychosexual disorder would compel him to use that position of authority to try to force them into sexual activity." At a hearing before the Retirement System in 1991, Brown conceded that Rizzo "hadn't admitted to any of the behavior for which he had been fired. . . . *His denial was part of his psychological disorder.*" The Virginia Supreme Court upheld Rizzo's claim that "he had a *'psychosexual disorder' that made him unable to supervise women without trying to coerce them into having sex with him,*" and ordered the state to pay Rizzo "a pension of $3,164 a month, with future cost-of-living raises. . . . The Virginia Retirement System also had to give him more than $200,000 in back payments dating to 1989, when the dispute began."[47]

Similar stories abound in magazines and newspapers. Larry Feldstein, a former New York City high school teacher, collects $3,300 a month tax-free in a disability pension, yet "bills himself as a skilled and graceful ski pro who can execute the 'perfect turn.' On a Mount Snow (Vermont) Web site, Feldstein calls himself a 'Perfect Turn Ski Pro who is also a certified senior fitness trainer.'" Feldstein retired in 1994 as a swimming and physical education teacher and was granted a disability pension, ostensibly because he had suffered a neck injury while demonstrating a hockey shot in April 1992. Three doctors on the system's medical board approved the disability."[48]

There is truth in the adage that what the state pays for, it gets more of. After centuries of punishing mental illness with deprivation of liberty, in the 1960s the state began to call mental illness "psychiatric disability" and undertook to reward it with disability payments. This policy has resulted in a hyperinflation of mental diseases, or, more precisely, of diagnoses of psychiatric disorders, useful for justifying claims for psychiatric disability.

OBTAINING THE NECESSITIES OF LIFE

There are only three ways that a person can obtain the necessities of life:

- As a producer, working, earning money, providing for his own needs by means of voluntary exchange with others; this is called "commerce."
- As a predator, using force or the threat of force to rob others of the goods and services he wants; this is called "crime."[49]
- As a parasite, dependent on others—parents, family, church, state—for food, shelter, and money; this may be called "extraction by need."[50]

An individual who does not want to be, or cannot be, a producer, must become a predator or a parasite or perish. Anything that discourages or prevents peaceful market relations among productive adults—regardless of whether it is due to biological, cultural, economic, medical, personal, or political factors—encourages predation or dependency or both. Often, the two coexist: many people we consider disabled and/or mentally ill engage in *de facto* predatory behavior, while many others use their dependency coercively in a quasi-predatory fashion. In short, there is nothing mysterious about the supposed connection between crime and mental illness. Mental illness is not a cause of crime; it seems that way because we attribute mental illness to many people who engage in lawless behavior.

Like most words describing human behavior, the terms "producer" and "parasite" carry a heavy load of emotional baggage.[51] It must be kept in mind that being a producer is not synonymous with being a good person, and being a dependent is not synonymous with being a bad person. "America's elite education," Davidson and Rees-Mogg write, "is more adept at training persons to redistribute income than to produce it. . . . In 1990, there were more lawyers in the United States than all the rest of the world combined."[52] Although many lawyers and most politicians (many of whom are lawyers) are income redistributors, they are, nonetheless, "producers." And so, too, are persons whose job is to incarcerate individuals whose crime is engaging in voluntary exchanges with others who wish to purchase (illegal) drugs.

"Producer" and "parasite" are not simply honorific and dishonorific terms; they have valid descriptive content. Regardless of what he does, the person who is economically self-supporting is a producer: he may be a farmer growing wheat or a psychiatrist treating imprisoned drug addicts. Similarly, regardless of why a person is nonproductive, the person who is economically dependent on others is a parasite: he may be a cherished infant or an able-bodied welfare recipient. Disease does not automatically annul the ability to be productive.

The Americans with Disabilities Act (AWDA) and Mental Illness: Rhetoric and Reality

The phenomena we call "disabilities" and those we call "mental illnesses" are both existential-vocational problems, *par excellence*. Both concepts are self-validating. As long as people believe that mental illnesses are diseases *that cause disability, against the will of the disabled person,* the twin illusions of disability and mental illness as, *ipso facto,* diseases will remain impregnable. This makes the AWDA an especially important source for pharmacratic social regulations.

One of the declared *political* aims of the AWDA is "to diminish the stigma of mental illness and reduce discrimination involving . . . at least 60 million Americans, between the ages of 18 and 64, [who] will experience a mental disorder during their lifetimes."[53] How do lawmakers know what counts as a mental disorder? They know it the same way psychiatrists know it: they decide. Having chosen to recognize mental illnesses as *bona fide* diseases, legislators proceeded to decide which of them were covered under the AWDA, and which were not, in effect creating two lists of mental illnesses, one congressionally accredited, another congressionally unaccredited. For example, claustrophobia and personality problems are covered, but kleptomania and pyromania are not. The APA recognizes both as mental disorders.[54]

Whatever might have been the avowed aim of the AWDA, its actual function is that of a judicial-political instrument for bestowing the largesse of the therapeutic state on some people, and withholding it from others.[55] For example, in 1999, the Supreme Court used the AWDA to promote transferring mental patients from large state hospitals to so-called group homes, a brutal charade officially called "deinstitutionalization" but actually a form of transinstitutionalization. "Isolating people with disabilities in big state institutions when there is no medical reason for their confinement," declared the Justices, "is a form of discrimination that violates federal disabilities law." Ira Burnim, the legal director of the Bazelon Center for Mental Health Law, praised the decision: "This is the first time the court has announced that needless institutionalization is a form of discrimination." Curtis Decker, executive director of the National Association of Protection and Advocacy Systems, called the decision a "touchstone for the disability community" and said it would provide "a strong incentive for states to continue the trend toward deinstitutionalization."[56] Thus does moving psychiatric slaves from one plantation to another become another advance in psychiatry and civil rights.[57]

In modern mass democracies, laws and regulations based on concepts such as disability and mental illness are largely the tools of statist politicians busying themselves with redistributing income to guarantee "social justice." When lawmakers combine disability and mental illness, the result may still be called "law," but it ceases to be the rule of law. Brian A. McLaughlin, a Canadian attorney, examined the way courts deal with people claiming disability benefits due to mental illness. He noted that "the plaintiff will present expert medical evidence to the effect the plaintiff is mentally ill, and the defendant will present medical expert medical evidence saying the plaintiff is not mentally ill," and asked, "How, then, does the court decide which medical evidence to accept?"[58] He concluded: "The real question is whether the judge is prepared to accept the argument that the plaintiff is *not responsible* for his or her behavior. . . . Behind the facade created by the medical expert witnesses, such cases are not decided on medical grounds at all. . . . The real issues in such cases are not medical, but moral."[59]

Medical and psychiatric experts reject such a simple but unpalatable truth. Declares Kessler: "The cancer of workmen's compensation is litigation."[60] Kessler prefers giving even more power to doctors, ignoring that litigation is as intrinsic to a democratic system of disability compensation as voting is to a democratic system of elections. If certain persons are deemed to be entitled to monetary payment because they are disabled, then there must be persons and procedures to determine who qualifies and who does not. In the final analysis, the interest of the recipient is to receive, and of the donor to withhold. How is the conflict resolved? It is resolved politically, by political premises and procedures made to appear as if they were medical.

When society was ruled by aristocrats, as in ancient Rome, Elizabethan England, or Wilhelmine Germany, the donors decided who should receive what and on what terms. When society is ruled by pharmacrats, as it is today in the United States, doctors, lawyers, and judges decide. Since the interests of donors and recipients conflict, there can be no completely satisfactory method of allocating disability benefits. Whatever is done, some people will believe that too many are receiving too much, and some will believe that too few are receiving too little. The aristocratic system, which treated benefits as a *charity* and beneficiaries as *moral failures,* favored the donors. The democratic system, which treats benefits as *entitlements* and beneficiaries as *hapless victims,* favors recipients.

THE DISABILITY INFLATION

There is little disability among people barely maintaining themselves in a subsistence economy. The disabled die. As people's economic situation improves, their health, as determined by objective medical standards, improves, and so does the incidence of disability, as determined by bureaucratic standards. Although the reasons for this are obvious, experts on health policy often ignore the inverse relationship between economic progress and disability. Medical advances enable increasing numbers of sick persons to survive, often for long periods. Economic progress enables society to support increasing numbers of unproductive persons. Attributing nonproductivity to mental illness further inflates the number of disabled persons. The result is a veritable disability explosion, in the United States as well as in Europe. The following statistics tell the story.

- Between 1960 and 1970, the number of Americans receiving long-term disability benefits rose "from about 3.7 million to about 6.7 million."[61]

- In 1968, 9.3 percent of the American labor force was on the "medical dole"; ten years later, the figure was 14.7 percent. The cost to employers of Workers' Compensation grew from $2.1 billion in 1960, to $57.3 billion in 1993, an increase of almost 3,000 percent.[62]

- Between 1968 and 1978, the percentage of persons receiving disability payments as a proportion of the labor force increased from 11.3 percent to 15.1 percent in Germany; from 4.4 percent to 13 percent in the Netherlands; and from 9 percent to 18 percent in Italy.[63]

These figures reflect, *inter alia*, the modern passion to deny the diverse but enduring manifestations of adult dependency and the urge to mask them as medical problems susceptible to medical solutions.

Fueling the Disability Inflation

In her book *The Disabled State*, Stone shows convincingly that there is no necessary connection between disease and disability. She acknowledges that "the difficulty of reconciling disability as a purely medical concept with disability as an economic (or vocational, social, and personal) concept stands out as the critical problem in contemporary evaluations of the program, and that disability benefits are increasingly awarded for those disorders that are hardest to assess . . . [that is,] mental as opposed to physical conditions."[64] Yet, she does not acknowledge that disease plays a minor role in the impairment of most persons on the disability rolls of modern societies and fails to connect the disability inflation with the political-psychiatric crusade *to make mental illness look like the real disease it is officially claimed to be*. This is the more astonishing as she correctly observes that when "ideology mandates that everyone should work but society cannot provide employment for large segments of the population, the dilemma can be resolved by *defining* a higher proportion of population as disabled."[65] This is true not only for persons for whom "society cannot provide employment," but also for those who occupy the disabled role rather than work. At the same time, the political-psychiatric ideology demanding parity for mental illness negates legislative efforts *to limit* disability compensation to persons suffering from job-related physical injuries or illnesses.

Experts acknowledge that the disability inflation is fueled largely by increasing numbers of persons being added to the rolls of patients considered disabled by mental disorders:

- "Mental illness is an important cause of disability for younger workers."[66]

- "Mental illness is an important cause of disability. In the SSI [Supplemental Security Income] and DI [Disability Insurance] populations, the number of individuals with a primary diagnosis of a mental illness has grown steadily during the past decade [1996–1997]."[67]

- "The growth in mental disorder awards is the expected consequence of a society finally reaching out to an underserved population."[68]

Many authors acknowledge that "disability is subject to ever more expansive classification and codifications."[69] The following is an example of such expansive classification.

Nick de Paoli has worked for the A&P Company for 32 years. "In 1994, facing pressure from grocery chain officials, he began working 70–hour weeks, lost 35 pounds, had severe trembling, heart palpitations and numbness in his left arm." Convinced he was having a heart attack, he went to the hospital, was given a diagnosis of panic disorder, and did not return to work for six months. He sued for worker's compensation. In February 2000, after a four-year court battle, the New York Court of Appeals ruled that de Paoli "was entitled to coverage by the state's workers' compensation program, *even though he did not suffer a physical injury. In its ruling, the court recognized that the psychiatric injury de Paoli suffered is just as eligible for coverage as a physical injury.*" Chief Judge Judith Kaye explained: "[Mr. de Paoli] was forced by A&P to work longer hours . . . and manage a store that was not performing well . . . [his] psychiatric condition was caused by ongoing job stress." De Paoli's attorney predicted that the ruling "will open the door" to other compensation cases based on psychiatric injury.[70]

Most people disabled by physical illnesses are rehabilitated and removed from the disability rolls, whereas most people disabled by mental illnesses are not rehabilitated and remain on the rolls for long periods.[71] Disability bureaucrats regard this discrepancy as a frustrating problem. I regard it as evidence that mental patients do not have diseases; instead, they occupy a social role, officially interpreted as due to a chronic illness and hence an entitlement for accessing housing and money. Once again, the differences between medical and mental illnesses and medical and mental patients are noteworthy.

- The typical medical patient is not considered dangerous to himself or others, lives in his own home or that of a family member, and is gainfully employed. He is called "ill" because he has a demonstrable disease, not to justify classifying him as entitled to disability benefits.

- The typical mental patient is considered dangerous to himself or others, has no home of his own, and is unemployed. Although he has no true disease, he is called "ill" to justify classifying him as entitled to disability benefits.

It is hardly surprising, then, that most disabled mental patients cannot be rehabilitated and that the number of such patients is steadily increasing. Stone is baffled: "There has been a *decrease in the rate of termination of disability pensions, either by death or by recovery.* . . . The meaning of this trend is unclear."[72] It is unclear only if we view mental illness as a true illness. It is clear if we view mental illness as a medical-legal fiction, created, in part, to enable adult dependents to qualify as disabled-by-disease; that understanding also dispels the mystery about the nonlethality of the disease and the patient's failure to recover from it.

Bracketing disability with disease is not only cognitively fallacious, it is also pragmatically unwise: it encourages treating disability as an unwanted condition that happens to a person against his will and thus obscures the element of responsibility for using the sick role for personal gain. Stone rightly traces the equation of illness with nonresponsibility for occupying the sick role to infectious diseases that "had little room for individual will or deception in its theory of causation." Such diseases were viewed as "a struggle between the virtuous human and the enemy microbe, in which society had to take the side of the human being."[73] It is a good analogy, but it must be used with caution. The issues of fault and responsibility may be relevant to the manner in which an infectious illness is acquired, as is the case with sexually transmitted diseases. The issues may also be relevant to the causation of injuries and illnesses, especially if they form the basis of disability claims and other types of tort litigation; in such cases we want to know whether the injury is due to the negligence of the other or the carelessness of the claimant or perhaps even his deliberate self-injury. Moreover, even in endogenous illnesses, such as diabetes or lupus, fault and responsibility may be relevant considerations, not for the presence of the disease itself, but for its competent management to prevent recurrences and disability. In such cases we need to know whether the patient's disability is due to the severity of his disease, his neglect of its proper treatment, or other circumstances.

Because health professionals believe in the reality of mental illnesses, they overlook the fact that as the number of mental patients incarcerated in mental hospitals decreased after the 1960s, the numbers of persons receiving disability for mental illness increased. Before the 1960s, most mental patients resided in mental hospitals and were supported by the state with room and board, much as children are supported by parents. (Prior to World War II, virtually all mental patients were hospitalized involuntarily, and only such patients were considered genuinely or seriously mentally ill.) Today, persons who *want* to enter a mental hospital are usually denied admission, and those hospitalized involuntarily are quickly discharged and given disability payments.[74]

CONCLUSIONS

In modern societies, physicians and other health-care professionals often act as certifying agents, that is, as intermediaries between the individual as patient-claimant, and the institution—typically the state—as a source of disability benefits.

Disability is a vocational-economic rather than a medical-therapeutic problem. Modern societies are characterized by a growing disposition to dispense disability benefits for mental disorders—a policy that distends the concept of diagnosis, disguises the true incidence of unemployment, and distorts the concept of disease.

5

PSYCHIATRIC MEDICINE
Disorder

Routine clinical experience teaches us that the overwhelming majority of schizophrenics are in the prime of physical health.

Manfred Bleuler (1972)[1]

Research in the last decade proves that mental illnesses are diagnosable disorders of the brain.

"White House Fact Sheet on Myths and Facts about Mental Illness" (1999)[2]

On the locked ward in the New York City program, [tuberculosis] patients have to agree to take their medications. No program should have the power to force pills physically down a patient's throat.

Editorial, *New England Journal of Medicine* (1999)[3]

Linguistically, mental illness is an illness, by definition. Although that concept is now virtually unchallenged, it rests on an uncritical use of language and a disregard for the operational meaning of the term "mental illness." As there is no egg in eggplant, there is no illness in mental illness. Yet, defenders of the psychiatric faith maintain that "mental illness is like any other illness."

DISEASE OR DISORDER?

The American Psychiatric Association (APA)—recognized by the American government, American medicine, and the American people as possessing the authority and competence required to define and classify mental diseases—periodically issues a document, titled the *Diagnostic and Statistical Manual of Mental Disorders,* listing the conditions officially recognized as *mental diseases.* In the Introduction to the fourth edition of the *Manual* (*DSM-IV*), the authors state: "Although this volume is titled the *Diagnostic and Statistical Manual of Mental Disorders,* the term *mental disorder* unfortunately implies a distinction between 'mental' disorder and 'physical' disorder, that is a reductionistic anachronism of mind/body dualism."[4] Allen J. Frances, professor of psychiatry at Duke University Medical Center and Chair of the *DSM-IV* Task Force, writes: "*DSM-IV* is a manual of *mental disorders,* but it is by no means clear just what *is* a mental disorder. . . . There could arguably not be a worse term than *mental disorder* to describe the conditions classified in *DSM-IV.*"[5] Why, then, does the APA continue to use this term? If the word "mental," as Frances says, "implies a mind-body dichotomy that is becoming increasingly outmoded,"[6] then we would expect a special catalogue of *mental* diseases to be phased out, not steadily enlarged. (Psychiatric physicians call the roster of maladies they diagnose and treat a *Manual of Mental Disorders*; nonpsychiatric physicians call their roster the *International Classification of Diseases.*)

Although etymological analysis cannot settle a controversial issue, it can show us where to look for clarification. I shall not belabor the view that the mind is not the brain, and hence cannot, according to the scientific definition of disease, be the location of disease.[7] Instead, I will begin by considering why psychiatrists classify *disorders* rather than *diseases.*

According to *Webster's,* the term "disorder," as verb, means "to disturb the order . . . disarrange." Not by coincidence, the words "disturbed" and "disturbing" are often attached to persons viewed as mentally ill. Until recently, these terms neatly captured the distinction between "neurotics," disordered in their own minds and hence considered "disturbed," and "psychotics," disturbing the public order and hence considered "disturbing." The idea that mental illness has to do with *disturbing the orderly functioning*—of the self, the family, the workplace, society—accounts for its traditional legal-psychiatric bracketing with dangerousness to self or others, and for the popularity of the belief that it is the psychiatrist's duty to control (treat) the alleged condition (illness) that (allegedly) causes it. As a noun, the term "disorder" refers to "a condition marked by lack of order, system, regularity, predictability, or dependability; . . . a breach of public order; disturbance of the peace of society; misconduct, misdeed . . . [also] sickness, ailment, malady." If mental disorders were conditions "marked by lack of order, . . . regularity, predictability," then they could not be classified, that is *ordered.* There are, in fact, certain *patterns of regularity* in which people are "disturbed" and "disturbing." The construction of a system of classification of mental disorders rests on the observation that a certain orderliness, regularity, and predictability does characterize the conditions (behavior patterns) classified as mental disorders. This is why it is important that we challenge the weasel term "psychiatric disorder," which enables psychiatrists *to simultaneously claim and disclaim* that they can objectively identify mental illnesses and predict a particular patient's dangerousness.

In short, the term "psychiatric disorder" is useful because it enables psychiatrists to waffle: "It" may be a disease, or may not be; may render the patient incompetent, or may not; may annul intentionality, but not necessarily; may cause dangerousness to self and others, but not always; and be an excuse for crime, and may not be. It all depends on the psychiatrists' *interpretation* of their so-called clinical observations. This discretion enables them—aided and abetted by other physicians, lawyers, politicians, journalists, and the general public—to transform personal, marital, moral, political, social, and spiritual problems into mental diseases.

The APA's *Diagnostic and Statistical Manual of Mental Disorders*

The primary function and goal of the *DSMs* is to lend credibility to the claim that certain (mis)behaviors are mental disorders and that such disorders are medical diseases. Thus, pathological gambling enjoys the same status as a disease as myocardial infarction. In effect, the APA maintains that betting is an action the patient *cannot control*; and that, generally, all psychiatric "symptoms" or "disorders" are outside the patient's control. I reject that claim as patently false.

The authors of *DSM-IV* further assert that "a common misconception is that a classification of mental disorders classifies people, when actually what are being classified are disorders that people *have*."[8] Then, perhaps in an attempt to forestall the criticism that the psychiatrist's paradigmatic interventions are *forensic*—civil commitment and the insanity defense—the authors add this disingenuous disclaimer: "*DSM-IV* is a classification of mental disorders that was developed for use in clinical, educational, and research settings. . . . When the *DSM-IV* categories, criteria, and textual descriptions are employed for forensic purposes, there are significant risks that diagnostic information will be misused and misunderstood."[9] This disclaimer is contradicted by the actual uses of psychiatric diagnoses, in the United States and the Western world generally.

When the authors of *DSM-IV* warn of the "significant risks that diagnostic information will be misused and misunderstood," they do not say whose interests they endanger—those of psychiatrists or of patients. This opacity is part and parcel of the authors' denial that classifying mental disorders serves a vast apparatus of justifications—to help the "patient" when the apparatus is enlisted on his behalf and, more often, to harm him when it is used against him. The practical impact of the *DSM* on personal behavior and social, political, and economic policy can hardly be exaggerated: No psychiatric hospitalization or treatment, no claim for reimbursement for psychiatric services or psychiatric disability, no commitment order, no insanity plea is valid unless it is supported by an appropriate *DSM-IV* diagnosis.

The view that psychiatric diagnoses are the names of "neurobiological diseases," treatable with drugs, is now a defining element of what counts as correct psychiatric practice. In the 1999 Annual Report of the Ely Lilly Company, Prozac, Zyprexa, and Olanzapine are classed as drugs used for *"Neuroscience Disorders,"*[10] a remarkable honorific for chemical stimulants and straitjackets. Lilly's other products are categorized as drugs used in "Animal Health," "Diabetes Care," "Oncology," and "Primary Care." The terms "Science" and "Disorder" appear only in connection with psychiatric products. The disorders Lilly classifies as "Neuroscience Disorders" not only match the names of disorders listed in the *DSM,* but include "treatment resistant depression," evidently treatable—with a drug.

To validate the disease status of mental illness, psychiatrists resort to three overlapping claims, interpretations, or, perhaps most precisely, *strategies*. They are: (1) Mental illnesses are brain diseases. (2) Mental illnesses are "real" diseases, manifested by abnormal behaviors. (3) The term "disease" identifies the physician's perception of the patient's ailment, whereas the term "illness" identifies the patient's perception of it, in effect abolishing the possibility of distinguishing between sign and symptom, objective evidence of illness and subjective complaint. I shall briefly review the first and second views in this chapter, and consider the third, which pertains more to a philosophical than to a psychological analysis of the concept of disease, in the next chapter.

MENTAL ILLNESS IS BRAIN DISEASE

Psychiatrists maintain that our understanding of mental illnesses as brain diseases is based on recent discoveries in neuroscience, made possible by imaging techniques for diagnosis and pharmacological agents for treatment. This is not true. The claim that mental illnesses are brain diseases is as old as psychiatry.

Physicians often base their clinical diagnosis on the patient's appearance and behavior. For example, a patient may appear to be pale and complain of fatigue, and the physician may attribute the problem to anemia. The diagnosis of anemia will be confirmed or disconfirmed by laboratory tests; the diagnosis cannot be made solely on the basis of the patient's appearance and behavior.

Similarly, psychiatrists base their clinical diagnosis on the patient's appearance and behavior. For example, a patient may appear to be sad and his wife may report that he has threatened to kill himself, and the psychiatrist may attribute the problem to depression. Here the similarity ends. There are no objective diagnostic tests to confirm or disconfirm the diagnosis of depression; the diagnosis can and must be made solely on the basis of the patient's appearance and behavior and the reports of others about his behavior. The absence of objective diagnostic tests does not negate the validity of the psychiatric diagnosis; instead, the diagnosis affirms the validity of psychiatry as a medical specialty.

Mental Illness: A Medically Proven Disease

The assertion of modern psychiatrists that mental illnesses are brain diseases is, as I noted, not new. Benjamin Rush (1746–1813), the undisputed father of American psychiatry, wrote: "The subjects [mental diseases] have hitherto been enveloped in mystery. I have endeavored to bring them down to the level of all other diseases of the human body, and to show that the mind and the body are moved by the same causes and subject to the same laws."[11] John Thomas Arlidge (1822–1899), an English alienist, declared: "Can a man, imagining himself a king, or a millionaire, be physicked out of his delusion . . . ? . . . Is the delusion a freak of an immaterial something? If so, the notion that a dose of physic can repair the derangement may well be derided. But is it not rather the sign that a material, visible, and tangible organ or tissue is disordered; that a part of the man as material as his liver is unhinged, and that, like his liver, it is the seat of some morbid action, and just as much a subject for medical treatment?"[12]

Theodor Meynert (1833–1892), one of the founders of modern neuropsychiatry, began his textbook *Psychiatry* (1884), with this statement: "The reader will find no other definition of 'Psychiatry' in this book but the one given on the title page: *Clinical Treatise on Diseases of the Forebrain.* The historical term for psychiatry, i.e., 'treatment of the soul,' implies more than we can accomplish, and transcends the bounds of accurate scientific investigation."[13] Meynert postulated that mental diseases are brain diseases and predicted that psychiatry would merge into the study of the lesions of the frontal lobe and its connections.[14]

Meynert, Jean-Martin Charcot (1825–1893), and Karl Wernicke (1848–1905)—all of whom, incidentally, were Freud's teachers—were *neuropathologists.* They were mainly interested in the brains of deceased mental patients. Freud, too, began his career as a neuropathologist. When he took up medical practice, he was called a "*Nervenarzt,*" or "nerve doctor." It is not surprising, then, that these men used the *language of neurology and neuropathology* to speak about problems in living and blithely diagnosed persons displaying such difficulties as exhibiting the symptoms of nervous diseases.

In Freud's day, as now, one of the commonest neurological diseases was a stroke, often resulting in aphasia, that is, loss of the power to speak properly (motor aphasia) or to understand speech (sensory aphasia). When neurologists say that a person who had a stroke has "aphasia," they use the term literally. Some of Freud's early work dealt with this classic neurological syndrome. In his *Autobiographical Study*, Freud used the term metaphorically. Reminiscing about his days in Paris studying under Charcot, Freud noted that when he first arrived, Charcot ignored him. To endear himself to the Master, as Charcot was called, Freud offered to translate his lectures into German. "I can still remember a phrase in the letter, to the effect that I suffered only from '*l'aphasie motrice*' [motor aphasia] and not from '*l'aphasie sensorielle du français*' [sensory aphasia for French]. Charcot accepted the offer, and I was admitted to the circle of his personal acquaintances."[15]

Charcot was not only a great neurologist, he was also a medical guru and an accomplished actor. By the force of his commanding personality, the prestige of his office, the medical performances he orchestrated, the submission of his female patients, the assistance of his cowed subordinates, and the specialized terminology of neurology, he transformed the clerics' demonic possession into the clinicians' hysteria and pronounced it a genuine *brain disease*.[16] Freud saw through this charade and how well it served Charcot to achieve the fame to which Freud himself aspired. After returning to Vienna, Freud adopted Charcot's formula: Create a powerful neurological metaphor, treat it as if it were literal, and, *presto*, people flock to you as a Master of Diseases of the Mind. Soon, disciples will follow, whom you must bind to yourself by requiring them to perform the familiar rituals of ideological-semantic obeisance.

The view that mental symptoms are the manifestations of bodily diseases—in short, that the terms "mental illness" and "bodily illness" are synonyms, because all illnesses are *physical diseases*—was articulated forthrightly by the British psychiatrists Richard Hunter and Ida Macalpine. "When mental patients are investigated by modern methods," wrote Hunter in 1971, "mental symptoms are found to be epiphenomena which depend on type, rate of onset, localization and severity on the underlying disease process . . . the onus of being ill is [thus] *entirely* lifted off the patient who is the victim not of his mind but of his brain."[17] This is simplistic. We have a measure of responsibility for acquiring certain bodily illnesses, for example venereal diseases; and, as a rule, we have a measure of responsibility for recovering from treatable diseases.

Elsewhere, Hunter and Macalpine put their views thus: "Psychiatry is foremost a branch of medicine and subject to its discipline. *We do not accept that mental illness is somehow different from physical.* . . . Patients suffer from mental symptoms which like bodily symptoms are *caused by disease*. . . . Neurology which split off from psychiatry in the asylum's first decade established itself as a science when it became *anatomical*. Today enough is known of the brain to place psychiatry on *the same footing*."[18]

If we accept the proposition that X is not an illness unless there are *defining, objective, anatomical criteria for it*, in other words, that X is not an illness unless it can be diagnosed by examining some part of the patient's body, then it is absurd to call a condition that lacks precisely that characteristic a "real illness." It may happen in medicine that we do not yet know whether a problematic condition is or is not illness. This uncertainty is similar to the uncertainty in law about whether a defendant who seems to have committed a crime is or is not guilty. Faced with such a situation, we must proceed on the basis of an assumption or, as the law calls it, "presumption." Do we presume that the suspected condition is an illness and treat the subject as a sick patient? Or do we presume that it is not an illness and treat the subject as a healthy person?

In American law, a defendant is presumed innocent until *proven guilty beyond a reasonable* doubt. That is because being treated as guilty of a crime has deleterious consequences for the subject. Accordingly, our legal maxim proudly proclaims that it is better to let a thousand guilty persons go free than to convict a single innocent person. In American medicine, and in medicine generally, a person—especially if he or his relatives insist that he is sick—is presumed to have an illness and immediately becomes a *patient*; even if he is proven healthy beyond any reasonable doubt—by physicians ruling out all "organic illness"—he is considered sick, that is, mentally ill. That is because being treated as sick is believed to have beneficial consequences for the so-called patient, while being treated as healthy is believed to have deleterious consequences for him. Accordingly, our medical maxim is that it is better to falsely diagnose and unnecessarily treat a thousand healthy persons than to mistakenly declare a single sick person healthy and thus deprive him of treatment (which may save his health or even his life). This violates the classic medical-ethical principle, "First do no harm," which is roughly analogous to the legal-ethical principle of presuming innocence. (Yet we continue to be surprised that our health-care costs keep rising and that this process seems beyond our control.)

Satisfied with the belief that the mind *is* the brain and that psychopathology *is* somatic pathology, contemporary psychiatrists ignore such considerations. The truism that both living and dead bodies have brains but only living persons have minds cuts no ice against this dogma, essential for the well-being of psychiatry. Nancy C. Andreasen, professor of psychiatry at the University of Iowa, asserts: "What we call 'mind' is the expression of the activity of the brain."[19] Samuel B. Guze, professor of psychiatry at Washington University in St. Louis, states: "The conclusion appears inescapable to me that *what is called psychopathology is the manifestation of disordered processes in various brain systems that mediate psychological functions.*"[20] Donald F. Klein, professor of psychiatry at Columbia University, and Paul H. Wender, professor of psychiatry at the University of Utah, write: "Biological depression is common—in fact, depression and manic-depression are among the most common *physical disorders* seen in psychiatry."[21]

What psychiatrists *do* conflicts glaringly with such claims. Pathologists examine cadavers, biopsy specimens, and body fluids. Surgeons operate on patients and repair or remove diseased parts of the body. Psychiatrists do not even perform physical examinations: they listen and talk to patients, ask psychologists to administer pencil-and-paper tests to them, give patients diagnoses and drugs, and certify them as fit for civil commitment or unfit to stand trial. Their claim that they treat brain diseases is manifestly absurd.[22]

In the end, we come down to the meaning of the term "mental illness": If we use it to mean brain disease, then psychiatry would be absorbed into neurology and disappear, as Meynert believed it would and should. However, pyromania is plainly not like multiple sclerosis, and treating a patient with schizophrenia without his consent is plainly not like treating a patient with anemia with his consent. Psychiatry is not about to be absorbed into neurology.

The insistence of contemporary psychiatrists that mental diseases are brain diseases has brought us full circle, reprising the views of some nineteenth-century psychiatrists. Ironically, they recognized that the human experiences called "mental illnesses" were metaphorical diseases and that the cure of souls called "psychotherapy" was a metaphorical treatment. In 1845, the Viennese psychiatrist Ernst von Feuchtersleben (1806–1848) wrote: "The maladies of the spirit (*die Leiden des Geistes*) alone, *in abstracto*, that is, error and sin, can be called diseases of the mind only *per analogiam*. They come not within the jurisdiction of the physician, but that of the teacher or clergyman, who again are called *physicians of the mind (Seelenärzte) only per analogiam.*"[23]

Emil Kraepelin (1856–1927), the creator of the first modern psychiatric nosology, and Eugen Bleuler, who coined the term "schizophrenia," both recognized that the diseases psychiatrists diagnose and treat may not be real diseases. In his classic, *Lectures on Clinical Psychiatry* (1901), Kraepelin stated: "The subject of the following course of lectures will be the Science of Psychiatry, which, as its name [*Seelenheilkunde*] implies, is that of the treatment of mental disease. It is true that, in the strictest terms, we cannot speak of the mind as becoming diseased [*Allerdings kann mann, streng genommen, nicht von Erkränkungen der Seele sprechen*]."[24] Similarly, in his classic *Dementia Praecox or the Group of Schizophrenias* (1911), Bleuler acknowledged: "It is not yet clear just what sort of entity the concept of dementia praecox actually represents. . . . Schizophrenia cannot easily be distinguished from malingering."[25]

However, reservations about mental illnesses not being true diseases were overcome by the medical, legal, and social needs to validate psychiatrists as real doctors, psychiatric confinement as real treatment, and persons incarcerated by psychiatrists as real patients. Psychiatrists had no other choice. Denying the validity of mental illness as disease negates the *moral legitimacy* of involuntary psychiatric interventions, the *medical legitimacy* of voluntary psychiatric interventions, and the *economic legitimacy* of psychiatric interventions as treatments. As in a theocracy authorities cannot afford to doubt the reality of God, so in a pharmacracy they cannot afford to doubt the reality of mental illness. Faith in the dominant fiction must be regularly reaffirmed by appropriate rituals. The psychiatrists' disease-affirming rituals have varied from time to time. Today, psychiatrists proclaim the reality of mental illness by worshiping at the altar of neurobiology and psychopharmacomythology, and by speaking the language of brain disease, chemical imbalance, neurotransmitters, and psychopharmacology. In fact, the history of psychiatry from 1850 to the present is essentially the history of changing psychiatric fashions—from neuropathology to psychoanalysis to psychopharmacology. Modern societies need psychiatry. A world without mental illness seems to frighten people, especially people who pride themselves on their disbelief in God.

Although psychiatrists and their supporters maintain that mental illnesses are brain diseases, they actually no longer rest their claims for psychiatry's power to cure disease or control dangerousness on adducing evidence of demonstrable pathological lesions, subject to verification and falsification. Instead, they base their claims on the authority of medical experts and political leaders, supported by "biological markers" of abnormal brain activities, exemplified by images obtained by means of positron emission tomography (PET) and other imaging techniques. However, even if the claim that a particular mental illness is the manifestation of a true brain disease were valid, it would establish only the presence of a new brain disease, not the validity of the concept of mental disease. That is what happened when certain types of madness suspected of being manifestations of brain diseases were shown to be *proven brain diseases*: for example, paresis and epilepsy ceased to be mental diseases and became instead infectious and neurological diseases. Moreover, if proven brain diseases do not justify the insanity defense and involuntary confinement or treatment, why should we accept putative brain diseases as justifications for such measures?

Mental Illness: A Politically Proven Brain Disease

In the nineteenth century, pathologists defined what counted as disease. Today, politicians often perform this function, especially with respect to the diseases we call "mental." The first president to take it upon himself to validate the disease status of mental illness was John F. Kennedy. In a message to Congress in 1963, he declared: "I propose a national mental health program to assist in the inauguration of a wholly new emphasis and approach to the care of the mentally ill. . . . We need . . . to return mental health care to the mainstream of American medicine."[26] At a White House Conference on Mental Health in 1999, President William Jefferson Clinton was more specific: "Mental illness can be accurately diagnosed, successfully treated, just as physical illness."[27] There was a chorus of consensus. Tipper Gore, President Clinton's Mental Health Advisor, emphasized: "One of the most widely believed and most damaging myths is that mental illness is not a physical disease. Nothing could be further from the truth."[28] First Lady Hillary Rodham Clinton explained: "The amygdala acts as a storehouse of emotional memories. And the memories it stores are especially vivid because they arrive in the amygdala with the neurochochemical and hormonal imprint that accompanies stress, anxiety, and other intense excitement. . . . We must . . . begin treating mental illness as the illness it is on a parity with other illnesses."[29] Surgeon General David Satcher concluded: "Just as things go wrong with the heart and kidneys and liver, so things go wrong with the brain."[30] It does not seem to occur to the media or to people that there are no illnesses outside of the realm of the mental health field whose disease status requires defense by the White House.

The view that so-called mental problems stand in the same relation to brain diseases as, say, urinary problems stand in relation to diseases of the kidney is superficially attractive, even plausible. The argument goes like this. The human body is a biological machine, composed of parts, called organs, such as the heart, the lung, and the liver. Each organ has a "natural function" and when this fails, we have a disease, such as coronary atherosclerosis, emphysema, hepatitis. If we define human problems as the symptoms of brain diseases, then they are brain diseases, even in the absence of any medically ascertainable evidence of brain disease. We can then treat mental diseases as if they were brain diseases.

The error in this reasoning is that if we add up all our body parts, the sum is obviously greater than its parts combined. A living human being is not merely a collection of organs, tissues, and cells; he is a person or moral agent. At this point the materialist-scientific approach to understanding and remedying its malfunctions breaks down. The pancreas may be said to have a natural function. But what is the natural function of the person? Devoutly religious persons and atheists have lungs and livers so similar that one may be transplanted into the body of another without altering his personal identity, but their beliefs and habits differ so profoundly that they often find it difficult or impossible to live with one another.

What is the natural function of the person? That question is like asking, How should we live? What is the meaning of life? These questions are religious-philosophical, not scientific-technical. That is why different religions, different cultures, and different persons offer different answers. The diversity of human values is no more surprising than is the diversity of, say, human language or custom.[31] Tolstoy put it unforgettably when he wrote: "All happy families resemble one another; every unhappy family is unhappy in its own fashion."[32]

We view the nature of *things,* living and nonliving, as teleologically determined: in the case of elements, by cosmic-physical processes; in the case of living beings, by biological-evolutionary processes; and in the case of artifacts, by human beings. Accordingly, we think of their *normative* attributes as residing in their nature: that is why we can *discover* them. However, we view persons as partly self-made, shaping their own goals and functions and thus modifying their very natures. From such an existential viewpoint, the *norms of being human* reside partly in nature, partly in persons (societies, cultures); in part, we discover them; in part, we create or invent them. Isn't that what we mean when we speak of "progress," especially moral progress?

When the physician enters the realm of the meaning of life and the control of personal conduct, he ceases to be a biological scientist. Instead, he dons the robes of the priest, the politician, the judge, the prison warden, and even the executioner, determining the legitimacy of moral values, judging the permissibility of personal conduct, punishing misbehavior, and so forth—all in the name of the *health* of the patient, the community, society, the nation, even mankind. We tend to forget that the title or training of the person designated to deal with a problem often defines the nature of the problem and the way its solution is perceived. (If your only tool is a hammer, everything looks like a nail.)

Although viewing medicine as a moral and political-economic enterprise does not require the technical sophistication necessary for understanding medicine as a materialist science, progress in this area has lagged, and continues to lag, far behind. Such progress requires a more critical understanding of medicine by philosophers and politicians, such as was displayed by Kant and Jefferson, instead of blind reliance on politically vetted medical experts, such as is displayed by contemporary philosophers and politicians.

The main reason why the public, the media, and even many scientists fail to understand the problems uniquely characteristic of and intrinsic to psychiatry lies in the psychiatrist's being *mandated* by society to fulfill multiple, often contradictory social roles: He is viewed and accepted as a neuroscientist, studying the brain; a neurologist, treating patients with brain diseases, with their consent; a mental health professional, treating patients with mental diseases, with or without their consent; a public health physician, protecting society from dangerous mental illnesses and dangerous mental patients; a philosopher and judge, deciding who has free will and responsibility for his actions and who has not, who should be punished and who should be "treated"; a guardian of incompetent persons, with power to decide every detail of his ward's life; and a prison administrator and jailer, managing institutions for the confinement of persons deemed "dangerous to themselves or others." No physician, no priest, no lawyer, no one else but the psychiatrist has this much power over other human beings.

To justify his power, the psychiatrist ought to have to explain why society entrusts him, and only him, with powers so extensive and discretionary, and why he rejects Jesus' injunction: "Render unto God what is God's, and unto Caesar what is Caesar's." Specifically, the psychiatrist would have to justify why, in conflicts between individuals, he is willing to represent the interests of both parties. Instead of attempting to offer such a justification, psychiatrists defend their power to coerce and excuse by defining it as "beneficence." James L. Levenson, professor of psychiatry at the Medical College of Virginia, characterizes psychiatry's mandate thus: "Psychiatrists and other mental health professionals are charged by society with a *mission* to relieve the suffering of mental illness. . . . We have a *collective responsibility* to prevent harm and to prevent needless suffering and death. This obligation is what ethicists call the duty of beneficence." The term "collective responsibility" is a euphemism for legally legitimized violence against persons called "dangerous" ("mental patients"). In the official psychiatric view, locking up people who have not been convicted of any crimes and drugging them against their will are virtuous actions—helping people "to be free from dehumanizing disease."[33] Coerced patients disagree.

Psychiatry and the Problem of Dangerousness

Overtly, the psychiatrist is a physician, a medical specialist; his medical identity is well recognized and not disputed. Covertly, the psychiatrist is a judge and a jailer; his penological identity is not well recognized and is often disputed and even denied. However, it does not require a semantic autopsy on the word "dangerous" to recognize that by so qualifying a person, we stigmatize and cast him out of society. We regularly use the adjective "dangerous" in lieu of the injunction "avoid!"—as in calling high-tension wires "dangerous."

I have shown elsewhere that it is legally and morally absurd to equate and commingle dangerousness to self with dangerousness to others and that the practice of delegating to psychiatrists the task of forcibly protecting persons from being dangerous to themselves or others opens a Pandora's box of problems.[34] Suffice it to add here that law and medicine are equally complicit in uncritically accepting the rhetoric of dangerousness as a justification for psychiatric coercions, especially coerced "treatments." We use the term "dangerousness" as a medical-legal-rhetorical gambit: persons who hallucinate are considered dangerous, can be incarcerated, and can be treated against their will, but persons infected with the HIV virus are not considered dangerous, cannot be incarcerated, and cannot be treated against their will.

Patients with infectious tuberculosis are more dangerous, and more demonstrably dangerous, to others than are mental patients. Yet, physicians have very narrowly limited powers to confine such persons, and *no powers whatever to treat them against their will.*[35] Because of an upsurge of tuberculosis in New York City in the 1990s, especially among homeless AIDS patients, the Commissioner of Health was authorized to issue "orders compelling a person to be examined for tuberculosis, to complete treatment, to receive treatment under direct observation, or to be detained for treatment."[36] (Only forty-four patients were detained on this basis in 1997.) The term directly observed therapy (DOT) refers to social workers or other health-care personnel visiting the patients wherever they live and ascertaining that they take the prescribed medications. They can reward compliance with food supplements, fast-food vouchers, movie passes, clothing, and money, but cannot impose penalties for noncompliance. In the United Kingdom, public health physicians proudly emphasize that no law in that country permits compulsory *treatment*:

- Section 37 of the UK's Public Health (Control of Disease) Act contains *"no power for compulsory treatment of [tuberculosis] patients. . . . [It] only allows for removal to a suitable hospital; the person is free to walk out of the hospital immediately."*[37]

- In fact, this section of the 1984 Act allows only for removal to hospital and "neither here nor elsewhere in current public health law is there any provision for compulsory treatment of patients. We would not like our clinical colleagues to be under the impression that the legal power to force patients to accept treatment exists."[38]

Despite this evidence, E. Fuller Torrey, an enthusiastic advocate of psychiatric coercion, claims that public health laws for controlling tuberculosis support the forcible *treatment* of schizophrenia patients: "Their tuberculosis could be *treated*, but not their schizophrenia. Is there something inherently different in brains and lungs? Or is it that our brains are not thinking clearly?"[39]

Patients with infectious venereal diseases are also more dangerous to others, and are more demonstrably so, than are mental patients. Nevertheless, physicians have no powers to confine them, let alone forcibly treat them. Such persons are free to infect anyone willing to engage in a sexual act with them and, according to the most up-to-date medical-ethical opinion, "Access to treatment for [women with] infertility should no longer be contingent on HIV status."[40] This despite the fact that the HIV virus is transmitted from the mother to the fetus.

Plainly, the terms "mental illness" and "dangerousness" have special justificatory functions in mental health law. In practice, neither has anything to do with the psychiatric control of unwanted persons. In the United States, the die was cast a hundred and fifty years ago. Ever since, American custom and law have endorsed the practice of locking up people in mental hospitals, regardless of whether they are demonstrably ill or demonstrably dangerous.

- In 1851, the State of Illinois enacted a statute that specified that "married women . . . may be received and detained at the hospital on the request of the husband of the woman . . . *without the evidence of insanity or distraction* required in other cases."[41]
- In 1997, in *Kansas v. Leroy Hendricks,* the U.S. Supreme Court declared: "States have a right to use psychiatric hospitals to confine certain sex offenders once they have completed their prison terms, *even if those offenders do not meet mental illness commitment criteria.*"[42]
- In February 2000, Wisconsin's oldest prison inmate, a ninety-five–year-old man, was "resentenced" as a sexual predator. A psychologist "testified for the state and said psychological tests performed on Ellefson indicated if he was given a chance, he would commit a [sex] crime. . . . After only minutes of deliberation, the *jury* found that Ellef J. Ellefson should be *committed for mental treatment* under the sexual predator law."[43] (Ellefson qualifies as a sexual predator. A young, sexually active, HIV-positive man who fails to so inform his partners does not.)

These practices prove that *de jure* the mental hospital system functions as an arm of the medical profession, but *de facto* it functions as arm of the state's law-enforcement system. Accordingly, I maintain that standard psychiatric practices do not represent *the abuses of psychiatry;* on the contrary, they represent *its "proper" uses,* sanctioned by tradition, science, medicine, law, custom, and common sense. The very definition of the word "certifiable" supports this interpretation of the psychiatrists role: formerly called "alienist," his job was, and is, to alienate, that is, remove, the subject from society: *Webster's* defines "certifiable" as "fit to be certified as insane, befitting an insane person."

The advocates of forcible psychiatric treatment are so convinced of the nobility of their cause, that they openly describe, on the NAMI website, how to incriminate a "loved one" by staging his dangerousness, so as to provide him with the treatment he allegedly needs:

Sometime, during the course of your loved one's illness, you may need the police. By preparing now, before you need help, you can make the day you need help go much more smoothly. . . . It is often difficult to get 911 to respond to your calls if you need someone to come and take your MI relation to a hospital emergency room (ER). They may not believe that you really need help. And if they do send the police, the police are often reluctant to take someone for involuntary commitment. That is because cops are concerned about liability. . . . When calling 911, the best way to get quick action is to say, "Violent EDP," or "Suicidal EDP." EDP stands for Emotionally Disturbed Person. This shows the operator that you know what you're talking about. Describe the danger very specifically. "He's a danger to himself "is not as good as "This morning my son said he was going to jump off the roof." . . . Also, give past history of violence. *This is especially important if the person is not acting up.* . . . When the police come, they need compelling evidence that the person is a danger to self or others before they can involuntarily take him or her to the ER for evaluation. . . . Realize that you and the cops are at cross purposes. You want them to take someone to the hospital. They don't want to do it. . . . Say, "Officer, I understand your reluctance. Let me spell out for you the problems and the danger." . . . *While AMI/FAMI is not suggesting you do this, the fact is that some families have learned to "turn over the furniture" before calling the police.* Many police require individuals with neurobiological disorders to be imminently dangerous before treating the person against their will. If the police see furniture disturbed they will usually conclude that the person is imminently dangerous. . . . THANK YOU FOR YOUR SUPPORT WHICH MADE IT POSSIBLE FOR US TO PROVIDE THIS INFORMATION TO THOSE WHO COULD BENEFIT FROM IT.[44]

MENTAL ILLNESS IS ABNORMAL BEHAVIOR

The term "mad-cow disease" refers to a fatal central nervous system disease of cattle, not to the affected animals' objection to their domesticated status. However, the term "mad killer," attached to a defendant charged with murder and diagnosed as schizophrenic, refers to his violation of the criminal law, not a disease of his central nervous system.

The person who views brain disease as a material entity or process and mental disease as a nonmaterial construct, and who nevertheless wants to defend the disease status of mental illness, faces a dilemma. Either he must conclude that the term "mental illness" is a metaphor or he must recast the definition of illness from biological terms to socioethical terms.[45] Many psychiatrists recognize that they do just that, but they do not acknowledge that by so doing they redefine the concept of disease.

Redefining Illness

Silvano Arieti (1906–1981), editor-in-chief of the prestigious *American Handbook of Psychiatry* and editor of the *World Biennial of Psychiatry and Psy-*

chotherapy, was recognized as one of the world's foremost authorities on schizophrenia. In his encyclopedic *Interpretation of Schizophrenia* (1974), he frankly acknowledged that schizophrenia counts as an illness only if we redefine the concept of illness. He wrote: "Can we state that schizophrenia is an illness? If we follow the concepts of Virchow . . . the answer is no. . . . If by disease we mean an undesirable state of the subject, resulting in alterations of his basic functions, including the psychological, then schizophrenia is certainly a disease. *Schizophrenia, as well as most mental illnesses or psychiatric conditions, does not the fit the medical (especially Virchowian) model.*"[46]

Today, psychiatrists are divided between those who endorse the scientific definition of disease and claim that mental illnesses are brain diseases, and those who reject or ignore that definition and instead boldly embrace criteria for what counts as illness completely unrelated to it. The views of Lawrie Reznek, author of *A Philosophical Defence of Psychiatry,* exemplify the latter approach. He writes: "Whether we ought to punish serial killers or treat them is not something that depends on the facts. . . . If we feel we ought to treat psychopaths, then they are ill. If we feel they should be punished, they are not. . . . It is our intuition that we ought to be treating depressive and schizophrenic murderers that leads us to classify them as ill and therefore not responsible. On the other hand, it is because of our intuition that we ought to be punishing Nazis that we do not classify them as ill."[47] In other words, Reznek proposes to replace the descriptive-biological concept of disease with a tactical-political concept of it, seemingly unaware that this method was popular in both Nazi Germany and the Soviet Union.

Redefinitions of the concept of illness, to make it fit mental illness, abound. Robert Kendell, professor of psychiatry at the University of Edinburgh, states: "By 1960 the 'lesion' concept of disease . . . had been discredited beyond redemption, but nothing had yet been put in its place."[48] Actually, many things have been put in its place, but none of the proposed definitions of disease can withstand critical scrutiny.

In 1979, George Engel, professor of psychiatry and medicine at the University of Rochester, proposed a New Medical Testament, which became popular among psychiatric Protestants. In a paper, titled "The Need for a New Medical Model," he proposed a "biopsychosocial model of illness," exemplified by "grief as a disease." Replacing pathology with psychobabble, he declared: "As with classic diseases, *ordinary grief constitutes a discrete syndrome* with a relatively predictable symptomatology. . . . It displays the autonomy typical of disease . . . a consistent etiological factor can be identified."[49] Engel's aim, which he did not conceal, was to medicalize mental illness and validate psychiatry as a medical specialty: "By obliging ourselves to think of patients with diabetes, a 'somatic disease,' and with schizophrenia, a 'mental disease,' in exactly the same terms, we will see . . . how concentration on the biomedical and exclusion of the psychosocial distorts perspectives and even *interferes with patient care.*"[50] This is a dangerous and ugly gambit: it distracts attention from the fact that real doctors do not use coercion to treat patients with cholecystitis, whereas mad-doctors typically use coercion to treat patients with schizophrenia. Surgeons welcome patients' seeking second opinions and require a signed consent form before they treat them, whereas second opinions and consent are the very antitheses of hospital psychiatric practice. Engel's rhetorical deception is typical of proposals to expand the category of disease to include mental illnesses.

In *Psychiatric Diagnosis*, Donald W. Goodwin and Samuel B. Guze write: "When the term 'disease' is used, this is what is meant: A disease is a cluster of symptoms and/or signs with a more or less predictable course. Symptoms are what patients tell you; signs are what you see. The cluster may be associated with physical abnormality or may not. *The essential point is that it results in consultation with a physician.*"[51] In this account, disease is a social relationship, a person seeking a "consultation with a physician," rather than an objectively demonstrable phenomenon. (It is an absurd view: if it were true, the absence of physicians would protect people from having diseases!) Goodwin and Guze's claim is inconsistent with the concept of disease as somatic pathology and is contradicted by the majority of psychiatrists who insist that *all* psychiatric diagnoses correspond to brain diseases.[52]

H. Tristram Engelhardt, Jr., professor of medical ethics at Baylor University, endorses a definition of disease so broad that it easily encompasses all mental illnesses, past, present, and future. "The concept of disease," he writes, "is used in accounting for physiological and psychological (or behavioral) disorders, offering generalizations concerning patterns of phenomena which we find disturbing and unpleasant."[53] Engelhardt's view of disease blends the physical with the psychological, making him conclude that "diseases such as asthma, cancer, coronary artery disease, etc., are as much psychological as pathophysiological" and that "mental deficiency, kleptomania, and paranoid reactions do count as diseases."[54]

Charles Rycroft, a leading British psychiatrist and psychoanalyst, recognizes that mental illnesses are *not* diseases, yet validates them as diseases because doing so is *useful*. He writes: "The neuroses resemble physical illnesses . . . but they are inexplicable without reference to the patient's personality and motives, i.e., *they are creations of the patient himself*. . . . The idea that the neuroses . . . are illnesses is a *useful social fiction* since it enables neurotic phenomena to be dealt with therapeutically, but it is based on a confusion of thought, viz., the equation of unconscious motives with causes."[55] Asserting that a neurosis, rather than a person, *has* symptoms is to treat a psychiatric abstraction as if it were a moral agent. This proposition is inconsistent with Rycroft's recognition that the patient's symptoms are "creations of the patient himself," in which case we ought to view the condition Rycroft calls a "neurosis" as a type of malingering, not a type of illness. Finally, the suggestion that viewing neurosis as illness is a "useful fiction" is tantamount to a confession of professional bankruptcy. It is an admission that, in psychiatry, the identification and classification of diseases serve the causes of professional expediency and psychiatric gnosticism—a gnosticism enabling the psychiatrist to enter into every aspect of life and unlock its mysteries.

Psychologists have their versions of illness and mental illness. For the most part, they ignore, or are ignorant of, the Virchowian concept of disease and propose instead definitions of illness and mental illness in terms of abstract verbal formulae, with no identifiable referents. Like psychiatrists, psychologists also sidestep the challenge of distinguishing between literal and metaphorical diseases. The following excerpts are but a small sample from a vast literature.

Jerome Wakefield, professor of social work at Rutgers, whose definition of disorder is often favorably cited in the psychological literature, states: "A condition is a disorder if and only if (a) the condition causes some harm or deprivation of benefit to the person as judged by the standards of the person's culture . . . and (b) the condition results from the inability of some internal mechanism to perform its natural function."[56] It is easy to see why this kind of verbal gymnastics is popular among *clinical* psychologists craving the power and prestige of physicians. Wakefield's formula not only severs the notion of disorder from connection with the body; it also replaces the clear criterion of anatomical lesion or physiological malfunction with the obscure criterion of "inability of some internal mechanism to perform its natural function."

Raymond M. Berger, professor of psychology at Illinois State University, acknowledges that "the prevailing state of affairs in the mental health field is one in which we have been unable to agree on a definition of our central concept, that of 'psychopathology' (or, synonymously, 'abnormality' or 'mental disorder'),"[57] and suggests that "functional impairment or *disability*, not the presence of a lesion, is the essential element in the medical concept of disease."[58] This is another blatant difference between the ways real diseases and mental diseases are said to exist. Many medical diseases, especially asymptomatic diseases, are not disabling.[59]

Peter E. Nathan, a professor of psychology at the University of Iowa, maintains that mental illnesses are diseases because "consensus exists on a definition of psychopathology. It is embodied in *DSM-IV*, used in this country by more than 500,000 mental health professionals."[60] Rule by the opinion of the greatest numbers.

In 1968, Karl Menninger, the undisputed leader of postwar American psychiatry, defined mental illness as "a certain state of existence which is uncomfortable to someone. . . . The suffering may be in the afflicted person or in those around him or both."[61] And in 1999, Leonard J. Duhl, professor of public health at the University of California, defined both mental illness *and* poverty as "the inability to command events that affect one's life."[62] Such is the end result of imperialist efforts to expand the concept of mental illness.

Mental Illness: A Disease *Sui Generis*

The suspicion that, in the final analysis, mental illness is a disease *sui generis,* unique among diseases, is confirmed by the fact that it is the only disease believed to be capable of *causing and excusing crime.* In possessing this property, mental illness combines functions previously attributed to the Devil and God. Also, mental illness is the only disease that justifies, as "hospitalization," the preventive detention of persons deemed "dangerous to themselves and/or others" and the incarceration of persons deemed to be "sexual predators" who have served their prison sentences.

Psychiatrists, psychologists, philosophers, politicians, and others who labor to assimilate mental illness to body illness systematically fail to acknowledge that an intrinsic function—I would say primary function—of the mental hospital has always been the psychiatric segregation and control of unwanted persons, justified by their alleged dangerousness to themselves and/or others. This contention is confirmed by the whole history of psychiatry; the so-called psychiatric abuses in National Socialist Germany and the Soviet Union; and the continued popularity, in the West, of psychiatric rationales and facilities for imprisoning individuals whose detention cannot be justified as punishment for crime.[63] Recent opinions by Justices of the Supreme Court amply support this interpretation.

In 1992, in *Foucha v. Louisiana*, Justice Clarence Thomas asserted that it is constitutional to confine a "sane but dangerous insanity acquittee." Why? Because "unlike civil committees, who have not been found to have harmed society, insanity acquittees have been found in a judicial proceeding to have committed a criminal act. . . . In this very case, the panel that evaluated Foucha in 1988 concluded that there was '*never* any evidence of mental illness or disease since admission.' The trial court, of course, concluded that Foucha was 'presently insane,' at the time it accepted his plea and sent him to Feliciana [a forensic psychiatric institution in Louisiana]." Thomas concluded that "although his [an insanity acquittee's] mental disease may have greatly improved, he may still be dangerous because of factors in his personality and background other than mental disease. Also, such a standard [permitting involuntary mental hospitalization of a sane person] provides a means for the control of the occasional defendant who may be quite dangerous but who successfully feigned mental disease to gain acquittal."[64]

Let us keep in mind that physicians cannot treat competent adults without their consent; cannot treat (incompetent) minors without the consent of their guardians (typically, the parents); and cannot treat incompetent adults (disabled by medical illness) without the consent of their guardians (chosen by the patients in advance directives or appointed by courts). The guardians of *medical patients* are *never* the physicians who treat them. In medical practice, treatment decisions for *incompetent patients* are made by their guardians, not their physicians. By contrast, in psychiatric practice, *competent patients* are routinely treated against their will and treatment decisions are routinely made for them by their treating psychiatrists (whose decisions are, if necessary, routinely rubber-stamped by judges).

Sooner or later we must confront the glaring *disparity* between the legal status of medical and mental *patients*.[65] This disparity is usually justified on the ground that medical diseases, unlike mental diseases, are unlikely to impair the patient's competence to elect or reject treatment. Patients with sarcoma are assumed to remain in possession of their mental faculties, but patients with schizophrenia are not. Medical patients are therefore treated as contracting moral agents; medical hospitals and (nonpsychiatric) physicians do not physically prevent patients from leaving medical hospitals, and hence are never accused of imprisoning them. (The temporary restraint of a delirious—for example, postoperative—patient differs so radically from the months-and years-long restraint of the mental patient that I reject the validity of an analogy between them.) Mental patients, however, are often treated as if they were minors or unconscious; mental hospitals and psychiatrists regularly prevent patients from leaving mental hospitals, and hence are often accused of imprisoning them.[66]

As long as we regard mental illness as a cause of crime, much as we regard the AIDS virus as a cause of HIV infection, established psychiatric practices will endure. Whenever a person factually guilty of committing a serious crime pleads insanity, the jury is asked to answer a stupid question, namely, what "caused" the defendant to commit his wrongful act: his self or his illness? If the former, then he is a guilty victimizer. If the latter, then he is an innocent victim. The question is badly framed. Regardless of whether a person is deemed sane or insane, a person has *reasons, not causes,* for his action. If we reject the actor's reasons as absurd, crazy, or meaningless, then we consider and call him mentally ill. That, however, hardly constitutes proof that his alleged condition caused him to commit the forbidden act. In short, the insanity defense combines and conflates two problematic aspects of mental illness: 1) What is it as a phenomenon? (2) Does it cause and excuse bad behavior?

For the sake of clarifying the issue before us, let us admit as true the erroneous claim that insanity is a brain disease. In that case it is similar, say, to parkinsonism or a stroke, brain diseases diagnosed and treated by neurologists. A brain disease may, indeed, be a cause. But a cause of what? Typically, of a *functional deficit*, such as weakness, blindness, paralysis. No brain disease causes complex, coordinated behaviors, such as the crimes committed by John W. Hinckley, Jr.

The insane person is, after all, a person, a human being. "The madman," as Gilbert K. Chesterton put it so memorably, "is not the man who has lost his reason. The madman is the man who has lost everything except his reason."[67] Only legal tradition and psychiatric-professional self-interest, not facts or logic, compel the law to frame the jury's task as a choice between deciding whether an insane defendant is bad or mad—guilty (by reason of free will) or not guilty (by reason of insanity). If a person guilty of assault or murder is deemed to be mentally ill, he should be sentenced for his crime, imprisoned, and offered treatment for his "illness"; that is, he should be dealt with just as we deal with the criminal who has diabetes or tuberculosis. Millions of people are said to be mentally ill, but most of them do not commit crimes.

THE ILLUSION OF MENTAL ILLNESS

As I have offered critiques of the idea of mental illness elsewhere, a brief summary must suffice here. It is an elementary principle of logic that one cannot prove a negative. One cannot prove the nonexistence of mental illnesses, just as one cannot prove the nonexistence of ghosts. One can only point out that a belief in mental illness as a disease of the brain is a negation of the distinction between persons as social beings and bodies as physical objects, in the same way that a belief in ghosts is the negation of the distinction between life and death. When we negate the distinction between physical objects and social beings, between bodies and persons, the concept of disease ceases to be limited to the dysfunction of cells, tissues, and organs and expands to include personal conduct. This enables persons deputized by the state as its agents (psychiatrists) and informants (family, teachers, students, employers) to transform any behavior they deem troublesome into a mental illness requiring psychiatric intervention. The result is an erosion of privacy, dignity, liberty, and responsibility.

The Conceptual Critique

If psychiatric diagnoses are the names of brain diseases, then they are literal or real diseases; if they are the names of (mis)behaviors, then they are metaphorical diseases or nondiseases. No one believes that love sickness is a literal disease, but nearly everyone believes that mental illness is. However, the contemporary Western mind-set is so thoroughly medicalized-psychiatrized that it is fruitless to demonstrate the logical-linguistic misconceptions inherent in the claim that "mental illness is like any other illness." Some philosophers have lamented the self-validating character of that claim. Ronald de Sousa, a professor of philosophy at the University of Toronto, observed:

> Suppose we accept the claim that the manifestations referred to as "mental illness" have biological causes, what would that entail about the existence of mental illness? The answer is *absolutely nothing*. For by exactly the same token the manifestations labeled "sane behavior" have biological causes. So what is the difference? The obvious suggestion is that the causes of mental illness consist in biological malfunction or organic sickness. . . . But actually, if we can show this we have done the opposite of what we intended: instead of vindicating the concept of mental illness we have rendered it otiose. For we now have an organic illness to worry about. . . . But now either mental illness is *reduced* to physical illness, or it refers to *symptoms* of physical illness. Neither alternative vindicates the concept.[68]

Conventional wisdom as well as political correctness preclude entertaining the possibility that mental illness, like spring fever, is a metaphor. Ordinary language is, of course, metaphorical through and through. "The greatest thing by far," declared Aristotle, "is to be a master of metaphor."[69] Conversely, being a willing slave of metaphor or using metaphor to enslave others constitutes an abuse of language, with grave consequences, typically for the speaker's intended victim, but in the end usually for the speaker as well.

Linguistic clarification, such as I have just offered, is helpful to persons who want to think clearly, regardless of consequences. However, it creates a conflict for persons who want to respect social institutions whose integrity rests on the literal uses of key metaphors; who want to have successful careers in those institutions; or, perhaps most importantly, who want to make use of the services offered by those institutions. Whenever someone invokes the term "mental illness," we must ask, *Cui bono*? (Who profits [from the stratagem]?) Many persons have family members whom they want to control by means of state-sanctioned, coerced psychiatric interventions. This is probably the main impetus for literalizing the metaphor of mental illness—lending credibility to the belief that mental illnesses are true diseases, *causing* the patient to be dangerous to himself and others, and *justifying* the interventions and institutions based on that belief.

Nowadays, we routinely give disease names not only to bodily diseases, but also to (mis)behaviors. There is a good reason for this. *If we want to treat a particular (mis)behavior, as a matter of law or social policy, as if "it" were a disease*, we are *expected* to call it a "disease," for example, "alcoholism." It is not surprising, then, that we diagnose mental illnesses by finding abnormalities (unwanted behaviors) *in persons*, not abnormalities (lesions) *in bodies*.

Unsurprisingly, the psychiatric establishment remains unconvinced by my views. Kendell dismisses my work with the following remark: "Szasz' famous jibe that 'schizophrenia does not exist' would have been equally meaningless had it been made in regard to tuberculosis or malaria. The organisms *Mycobacterium tuberculosis* and *Plasmodium falciparum* may reasonably be said to exist, but the diseases attributed to their propagation in the human body are concepts just like schizophrenia."[70] Kendell ignores that the diagnosis of malaria rests on demonstrating the presence of a parasite, and that the diagnosis of schizophrenia requires no similar evidence.

The Consequentialist Critique

The idea of mental illness may be broken up into two interrelated parts—a faulty conceptualization (failure to distinguish between disease and nondisease) and an immoral justification (rationalizing coercion as treatment). Accordingly, my critique of the concept of mental illness is two-pronged, one conceptual or philosophical, the other consequentialist or political. My conceptual critique is focused on the distinction between the literal and metaphorical uses of language; my political critique is focused on the distinction between dealing with persons as adults, responsible for their behavior, as against dealing with them as infants or idiots, not responsible for their behavior.

It is a fallacy to assume that persons called "patients" are sick, and vice versa. We must distinguish between being ill and being a patient, between having an abnormal biological condition called "disease" and occupying the social status called the "sick role." Although many sick persons are patients, and many patients are ill, it is obvious that a person may be sick and not be a patient, and that a person may be called a "patient" and not be sick.

The differences between the descriptive and prescriptive modes of language merit a brief comment here. Saying that John's hair is brown is a description; saying that he should have it cut is a prescription. A descriptive sentence is the report of an observation that asks nothing of anyone. A prescriptive sentence is a request for a specific response. Because psychiatrists have power over persons denominated as patients, their nominally descriptive statements typically function as covert prescriptions. For example, they may describe a man who asserts that he hears God's voice telling him to kill his wife as "schizophrenic":

This diagnosis functions as a prescription or mandate—for example, to hospitalize the patient against his will (lest he kill his wife) or, after he has killed her, to acquit him on the ground of insanity and hospitalize him against his will (lest he kill himself or others).

Ostensibly, what justifies the psychiatrists' use of force is the assumption—concealed in and intrinsic to the idea of mental illness—that the mental patient is legally incompetent and that coercing him is a form of treatment. These twin presumptions permit psychiatrists to pretend that coercion may, at any moment, be a necessary element in the conscientious and correct practice of their particular branch of medical healing. Because psychiatric coercion is defined as serving the best interests of coerced patients, both law and psychiatry regard the principle of eschewing psychiatric coercion as synonymous with "withholding lifesaving treatment" from patients who need it. As a result, when a person under the care of a psychiatrist kills himself or someone else, his psychiatrist may be judged guilty of medical negligence.

If we restrict the concept of treatment to a voluntary relationship between a medical practitioner and a competent client (or his legal guardian or proxy), then medical interventions against a patient's will are, *by definition,* not treatments. *In a free society, the physician's right to treat a person rests not on his diagnosis but on the subject's consent to treatment.* If we further restrict the concept of treatment, as we should, to interventions aimed at remedying a true disease, then medical interventions serving other purposes are, again *by definition*, not treatments. For example, cosmetic procedures performed by plastic surgeons, such as removing wrinkles, are *medical interventions but not medical treatments*, because they do not remedy a disease. Similarly, abortion, if the woman is healthy, is not a treatment, because a normal pregnancy is not an illness—albeit it may be an inconvenience in the life plan of the pregnant woman or of the man who impregnated her or both. To be sure, a surgical abortion requires anatomical, medical, and surgical knowledge and skill and is therefore a "medical intervention." However, the act does not transform pregnancy into a disease. Thus does our unwillingness to distinguish between complaints and diseases prevent us from distinguishing between medical interventions and medical treatments and create a host of other economic, ethical, and political problems as well.[71]

Linguistic considerations highlight some of the obvious differences between bodily disease and mental disease. If we speak English competently, we do not attribute motives to bodily diseases and do not call a motivated action a bodily disease: We do not attribute motives to a person for having leukemia; do not say that a person has reasons for having glaucoma; and would be uttering nonsense if we asserted that diabetes has caused a person to shoot the President. But we can and do say these things about a person with a mental illness. One of the most important philosophical-political features of the concept of mental illness is that, in one fell swoop, it detaches motive from action, adds motive to illness, and thus destroys the very possibility of separating disease from nondisease, and hence diagnosis from disease.

- Medical diseases are *discovered* and then given a name, for example acquired immune deficiency syndrome (AIDS).
- Mental diseases are *invented* and then given a name, for example attention deficit hyperactivity disorder (ADHD).

It is a crucial element of my critique of the idea of mental illness that I reject the contention that once a person is categorized as a mental patient, *ipso facto* his status as a moral agent is diminished or annulled. The typical mental patient is a conscious adult, possessing free will and responsibility, who has not been declared legally incompetent. Regardless of psychiatric diagnosis, he is entitled to liberty, unless he is convicted of a crime punishable by imprisonment; and if he breaks the law and is convicted of it, then he is guilty of a crime and ought to be punished for it. *Under no circumstances should a person profit from psychiatric excuses or suffer from psychiatric coercions.*

Remarks on the So-Called Abuses of Psychiatry

While nineteenth-century bacteriologists and pathologists labored in their laboratories looking for evidence of true diseases, psychiatrists had only to reach for their Latin dictionaries to discover evidence of mental illnesses. For example, in the 1840s, white physicians diagnosed runaway black slaves as mentally ill, suffering from "drapetomania" and "dysaesthesia Aethiopis."[72] (Since I first called attention to this diagnostic curiosity in 1971, it has become a part of the literature of psychiatric criticism.)

Toward the end of the century, finding diseases in the dictionary was raised to the level of a psychiatric art form by Baron Richard von Krafft-Ebing (1840–1902), a German-born psychiatrist who was professor of psychiatry, successively, at the Universities of Strasbourg, Graz, and Vienna. The work that made Krafft-Ebing world famous is *Psychopathia Sexualis*, the first edition of which appeared in 1886. Krafft-Ebing was an early practitioner of the art of transforming, with the aid of Latin and a medical diploma, behaviors considered sinful into sicknesses.[73] Modern sexology became an integral part of medicine—and the new science of psychiatry—simply by physicians' authoritatively classifying *sexual perversions* as "cerebral neuroses," and by lawyers, politicians, and the public embracing the transformation.

To impress the medical character of his work on the profession and the public, Krafft-Ebing sprinkled his text liberally with Latin, and he and his publisher alike maintained that *Psychopathia Sexualis* was written only for medical professionals, and solely for medical use. In the Preface to the first edition, Krafft-Ebing wrote: "The object of this treatise is merely to record the various *psychopathological manifestations of sexual life in man.* . . . The physician finds, perhaps, a solace in the fact that he may at times refer those manifestations which offend against our ethical and aesthetical principles to a diseased condition of the mind or the body."[74] I list, without further comment, some of the diseases Krafft-Ebing identified as "cerebral neuroses": "*Anaesthesia* (absence of sexual instinct) . . . *Hyperaesthesia* (increased desire, satyriasis) . . . *Paraesthesia* (perversion of the sexual instinct) . . . *Sadism* (the association of lust and cruelty) . . . *Masochism* is the counterpart of sadism . . . *Fetishism* invests imaginary presentations of separate parts of the body or portions of raiment of the opposite sex . . . with voluptuous sensations."[75]

Freud extended Krafft-Ebing's psychopathologizing of behavior from sexual behavior to everyday behavior. In *The Psychopathology of Everyday Life* (1901), he inverted Shakespeare's humanistic interpretation of conflict as an integral part of life into a dehumanized interpretation of tragedy as a manifestation of psychopathology.[76] Shakespeare displayed tragic figures, such as Hamlet, Lear, and Lady Macbeth, coping with conflicts. Freud showed us that their behaviors were manifestations of psychopathology. For Freud, as for Krafft-Ebing, unconventional sexual behaviors, especially masturbation, were manifestations of disease. But, unlike Krafft-Ebing, who limited himself to diagnosing only disapproved sexual acts as diseases, Freud went all the way, attributing normal behaviors as well to masturbation or some other "sexual noxa" and thus qualifying as diseases. The following list represents only a small sample of the products of his "scientific method."

- "Self-punishment is the final substitute for self-gratification, which comes from masturbation."[77] "Neurasthenia in males is acquired at the age of puberty. . . . Its source is masturbation."[78] "This second noxa is *onanismus conjugalis*—incomplete intercourse in order to prevent conception."[79] "Undoubtedly there exist cases of juvenile neurasthenia *without* masturbation, but *not* without the usual preliminaries of overabundant pollutions—that is, precisely as though there had been masturbation."[80] "The use of a condom is evidence of weak potency, being something analogous to masturbation, it is the continuous cause of his [the patient's] melancholia."[81] "Melancholia develops as an intensification of neurasthenia through masturbation."[82] "The insight has dawned on me that masturbation is the one major habit, the 'primary addiction,' and it is only as a substitute and replacement for it that the other addictions—to alcohol, morphine, tobacco, and the like—come into existence."[83] "What would you say if masturbation were to reduce itself to homosexuality?"[84]

Ignoring the massive history of the abuses of mental illness terms, psychiatrists continue to rationalize the construction of mental diseases. In our age of victimology, everyone has his own favorite victim group, usually members of his own race or religion, whose persecution they want to condemn by declaring it a mental disease. In 1986, Israel W. Charny, Ph.D., Director of the Institute of the International Conference on the Holocaust and Genocide, stated: "The awesome facts of the Holocaust render existing models and values of virtually all disciplines nearly meaningless. . . . *it is inconceivable that we reconcile ourselves to mental health concepts that do not define . . . the leaders and followers who execute mass murder as disturbed and abnormal.*"[85] Not to be bested in the victimology Olympics, Alvin Poussaint, a prominent black professor of psychiatry at Harvard Medical School, declares: "My position is that *extreme racism is a serious mental illness because it represents a delusional disorder. . . . And I think it's treatable.*"[86] It's payback time for drapetomania and dysaesthesia Aethiopis.

The "scientific control" of behavior based on the "science of psychiatry" is a gigantic confidence game which consists of transforming, by means of psychiatric jargon, what is perfectly obvious into what is impenetrably mysterious. Its inevitable result is a series of crimes against humanity, usually perpetrated by the *crème de la crème* of the profession.[87] In the 1940s and 1950s, some of the most prominent American medical institutions, psychiatrists, and psychologists were engaged in medical "experiments" that differed only in degree and scope from those engaged in by Nazi physicians experimenting on the inmates of concentration camps. Working in secret for the CIA, psychiatrists systematically poisoned people and used electric shock treatments to destroy their memories, ostensibly in an effort to discover methods of "mind control." Like all psychiatric "abuses," this massive criminal conspiracy against the public was quickly forgotten.[88]

As long as we have no historical-moral accounting and hence no collective memory for psychiatry's crimes against humanity—similar to the accounting and memory for the wrongs of Christianity recognized by the papacy, slavery recognized by the American people, and the Holocaust recognized by Germany and the Western world—no *ad hoc* criticism of psychiatric "abuses" will have any impact on the prestige and power of psychiatry and no criticism of the concept of mental illness will be persuasive.

The Mirage of Biological-Reductionist "Explanations" of Human Behavior

Asserting that all human behavior is "biologically caused"—that we eat *because* we are hungry—is true only in a very trivial sense. It does not explain what we eat, how we eat, or why we eat at particular times. Despite such an obvious shortcoming, explaining behaviors called mental illnesses by attributing them to pathological processes in the brain has never been more popular, nor has the propaganda to make psychiatric coercions seem like ordinary medical acts been more intense.

In January 2000, Bruce H. Price, Raymond D. Adams, and Joseph Coyle, prominent physicians from the departments of neurology and psychiatry at Harvard Medical School, published a position paper in *Neurology*, the official journal of the American Academy of Neurology. In a paper entitled "Neurology and Psychiatry: Closing the Great Divide," the authors declared: "All mental processes are ultimately biological. . . . The historical debates about mind versus brain, nurture versus nature, and functional versus organic, should be abandoned. . . . Schizophrenia, mood disorders, obsessive-compulsive disorder, panic disorder, addiction, and autism are now recognized as psychiatric disorders *with underlying biological abnormalities* . . . brain dysfunction in many psychiatric diseases . . . occurs at a subcellular level."[89]

Mark Twain remarked that Wagner's music is better than it sounds. The assertion that "all mental processes are ultimately biological" sounds better than it is. It is the principle that leads us to attribute suicide to depression, and depression to neurotransmitters—which is like attributing marriage to lust, and lust to hormones. If, as I noted, everything that happens to or is done by human beings is *biological*, then saying so is a meaningless truism. Attributing mental illnesses, such as addiction and panic disorder, to biological alterations occurring at a "subcellular level" is a parody of the denial of free will, choice, and responsibility.[90] Scientists require strict proof before they accept an *etiological explanation* for an infectious or neoplastic illness. Psychiatrists and the public uncritically accept unproven claims as an *etiological explanation* for mental illness.[91]

It is one thing to understand the misbehavior of a dog and control its behavior in a kennel. It is a very different thing to understand the behavior of a person, much less control him, especially in a society in which he possesses inalienable rights. The inability or unwillingness of the expert, whether physician or lawyer, to concede this difference is regularly accompanied by his inability or unwillingness to acknowledge the conceptual primacy of the person as moral agent, that is, the cognitive absurdity and moral impropriety of reducing a person to his bodily or mental functions.

There is something positively bizarre about the modern, reductionist denial of persons. To be sure, brains in craniums exist; and so do persons in societies. The material substrates of human beings or persons are, indeed, organs, tissues, cells, molecules, atoms, and subatomic particles. And so, too, are the material substrates of human artifacts, say a wedding ring. Scientists do not claim to be able to explain the economic or emotional value of a wedding ring by identifying its material composition; nor do they insist that a physicalistic account of its structure is superior to a cultural and personal account of its meaning. Yet, many modern philosophers, physicians, and scientists claim that they can explain choice and responsibility by identifying its material substrate, that "life can be explained in terms of ordinary physics and chemistry."[92]

It is possible that certain patterns of behavior now called "mental illnesses" may, at some future time, be causally correlated with neuropathological lesions, at a subcellular level. It is equally possible that certain patterns of normal behavior, such as being multilingual, may, at some future time, be causally correlated with neurological processes, at a subcellular level. If and when that will be the case, then the "pathological" conditions in question will be *diagnosable as diseases by objective biological methods,* just as anemia and hypothyroidism are so diagnosable. At that point, but not before, those conditions will qualify as *bona fide* medical diseases. Even then, however, I do not see how those facts, per se, would justify the involuntary treatment of persons suffering from the diseases or their being held not responsible for their crimes.

Instead of acknowledging and considering such problems, Price and his colleagues assume, as most Americans now seem to assume, that psychiatrists ought to have certain powers no one else has. They write: "What interventions can we best employ to rehabilitate the patient's brain and behavior? . . . Psychopharmacology? Neurosurgery, i.e., stereotaxic lesions or cell transplantation? . . . With the impending probabilities of our ability to genetically, medically, and socially engineer the human brain, core questions need to be addressed. Who should make the decisions?"[93]

Price and his colleagues find it easier to speculate about future psychiatric-ethical dilemmas than to confront the problem of justifying civil commitment and the insanity defense. We seem to have reached the point in the growth of the therapeutic state where psychiatrists, politicians, and lawyers no longer need to grapple with these issues. The subtitle of a 2000 "Special Report" in the prestigious *American Bar Association Journal* reads: "Should the government force treatment on the mentally ill?" The author acknowledges that "many of the untreated mentally ill simply shun attempts to help them" and then approvingly relates the case of man who, ostensibly to obtain mental health treatment for his brother, denounced him as "dangerous," even though he was not: "*'I said the magic words. I knew I had to do it.'*"[94] He adds, without disapproval, that "advocates of forced treatment—they prefer the term '*assisted treatment'*—say such laws, especially outpatient commitment, are essential tools to both curb violence and make the best use of [the] system."[95] Abolishing psychiatric coercions and excuses forms no part of the debate about mental health law.

Making Saints and Making Mental Illnesses

"The poet's pen," wrote Shakespeare, "gives to airy nothing . . . a name."[96] The psychiatrist's pen gives to certain (bad) people a name, *mad*—just as the priest's pen gives certain good people a name, *saint*. With less dramatic effect, everyone's speech engages in this kind of naming, with the result that, in Robert Reininger's (German philosopher, 1869–1955) words: "*Unser Weltbild ist immer zugleich ein Wertbild*" (Our view of the world is, at the same time, a view of [our] values).[97]

Mental illness and sainthood are both fictions, that is, fabricated products. One is manufactured by authoritative rhetorical acts of *malediction,* the other by authoritative rhetorical acts of *benediction.* In his book *Making Saints,* Kenneth Woodward describes the process by which the Vatican transforms persons from mortal humans into quasi-divine beings. The process rests on a belief in saints: "They [Catholics] pray to them, they honor them, they treasure their relics, they name their children and their churches after them. . . . Christianity is . . . unlivable without saints."[98] Similarly, the process of transforming human conflicts into mental diseases rests on a belief in mental illness: psychiatrists give certain behaviors medical names, write books about them, teach them in schools, treat them with drugs and electricity, and build hospitals to house their "victims." Modernity is unlivable without mental illnesses.

"To 'canonize,'" Woodward explains, "means to declare that a person is worthy of universal public cult. Canonization takes place through a solemn papal declaration that a person is, for certain, with God. Because of that certainty, the faithful can, with confidence, pray to the saint to intercede with God on their behalf. . . . Since 1234, when the right to canonize was officially reserved to the papacy alone, there have been fewer than 300 canonizations."[99] In recent years there has occurred a dramatic increase in the manufacture of saints (as well as of mental patients). In a single year, 1988, Pope John Paul II canonized 122 men and women—almost half as many as had been created in the previous seven hundred years.[100] In 2000, he created 27 new Mexican saints. "It is very important for [Mexican] national pride," explained a church historian.[101] Asked whether he thought the church was making too many saints, Cardinal Joseph Ratzinger—prefect of the Congregation of the Doctrine of the Faith and John Pope Paul II's closest adviser on theological matters—"acknowledged that the number of saints and blesseds had increased in the previous decade. . . . The Italians, in particular, interpreted the cardinal's remarks as . . . a confirmation of those critics of the church who have long ridiculed the congregation as a 'saint factory.'"[102]

Although Woodward writes as a believing Catholic, he recognizes that "there is a tendency, inside the congregation and out, to confuse the mysterious ways of God with the unnecessarily mystifying ways of the saint-making process. For members of the congregation, I suspect, this tendency is rooted in the theological assumption that they do not *make* saints, but only discover those whom God has raised up in our midst."[103]

The pretense that creating a new psychiatric diagnosis is an act of *discovering* a disease—that inventing a name is discovering a phenomenon, that a rhetorical trick is an empirical finding—underlies the entire apparatus of psychiatric nosology.

The Public Betrayed: The Corrupted Expert

A layman cannot distinguish an original Renoir from a good forgery, nor can he distinguish disease from what only looks like disease. In such situations people rely on *experts* to help them distinguish between what is real and what is fake, vouching for the genuineness of the authentic or declaring the fake to be counterfeit, and advising their clients accordingly. Such utter dependence on the expert invites his corruption, seducing or suborning him to validate as genuine what he knows or suspects to be a fake. This phenomenon has long been a part of the art world, where it is a well-recognized problem.[104] It has become a part of the Holocaust literature, where acknowledging its existence is virtually taboo.[105] And, of course, it is a phenomenon intrinsic to psychiatry—as I have shown long ago[106] and will briefly show again—where its presence is at once recognized and repudiated.

When an art collector plans to purchase a masterpiece, he depends on the dealer's vouchsafing the work's history or pedigree, called "provenance." When a respected dealer resorts to the practice of issuing false provenances, the result is a spectacular scam, forgeries fetching astronomical prices.

Similar acts of false authentication were perpetrated by several famous writers and moralists, driven, one might assume, by their ideological zeal to magnify the unmagnifiable evils of the Holocaust. Nobel Laureate Eli Wiesel's review of Jerzy Kosinski's *The Painted Bird,* in the pages of the *New York Times Book Review,* is an example. According to Kosinski's biographer, James Park Sloan, Wiesel "sanctified the book as an authentic Holocaust testament."[107] In fact, the experiences attributed to the child-protagonist—seemingly the author—were fabrications. Cynthia Ozick cogently observed that both Kosinski and Wilkomirski (about whom more presently), used fictitious stories "to symbolize, typify, exemplify, [and] allegorize" the Holocaust and thus "dilute and obscure, even . . . crush, its historicity."[108]

In 1995, "Binjamin Wilkomirski"—a.k.a. Bruno Doessekker, a man born and raised in Switzerland—published his famous confabulation, titled *Fragments,* mendaciously subtitled *Memories of a Wartime Childhood.*[109] Holocaust expert Daniel Goldhagen hailed *Fragments* as a masterpiece: "Even those conversant with the literature of the Holocaust will be educated by this arresting book."[110] Child saver Jonathan Kozol wrote: "All children—most importantly Holocaust children—are finally vindicated."[111] *Fragments* won the Jewish Quarterly Literary Prize in London, the Prix de Mémoire de la Shoah in Paris, the National Jewish Book Award in New York, and an award from the American Orthopsychiatric Association (AOA). In a brilliant criticism of the experts who validated Wilkomirski's lies as truths, Ozick wrote: "A psychologist [speaking for the AOA] stated: 'We are honoring Mr. Wilkomirski . . . as mental health professionals. What he has written is important *clinically*.' From this it would be fair to conclude that mental-health professionals care nothing for historical evidence, and *do not recognize when they are, in fact, acting politically*. If Mr. Wilkomirski is indeed a fabricator, then to laud him is to take a stand, politically, on the side of those who insist that the Holocaust is a fabrication."[112] The person who affirms false Holocaust memories and the person who denies the reality of the Holocaust play the same game: each regards his cause as so sacred that lying in its interest is a noble act. The lie is defined and justified as a "higher truth."

Like art dealers who issue false provenances or Holocaust experts who legitimize lies as truths—and, after they are exposed, dignify them as "false memories"—psychiatrists have a long history of *systematically validating fake diseases as real diseases,* and getting away with it. They get away with it because the psychiatrists' lies—unlike those of art forgers and Holocaust memory forgers—are useful for the family and, increasingly, for the state. Indeed, the single most important issuer of false medical provenances today is the U.S. government. In December 1999, Surgeon General David Satcher released a report according to which

- "22 percent of the population has a diagnosable mental disorder." False: the figure is 100 percent, because anyone can be "diagnosed" as having a mental disorder.

- "Mental illness, including suicide, is the second leading cause of disability." True, so far as suicide is concerned: dead persons are disabled.

- "One of the foremost contributions of contemporary mental health research is the extent to which it has mended the destructive split between 'mental' and 'physical' health." If true, why do Satcher and the NIMH persist in using the term "mental illness" and why do we have a National Institute of *Mental* Health?

- "Mental disorders are . . . legitimate illnesses . . . [even though they] are usually not defined by laboratory tests or physiologic abnormalities of the brain."[113] Mental disorders are legitimate diseases because *the government now defines what constitutes a legitimate disease*: Donna E. Shalala, Secretary of Health and Human Services, stated: "In fact mental illnesses are just as real as other illnesses."[114]

"An ambassador," said Sir Henry Wotton, a seventeenth-century English poet and diplomat, "is an honest man sent abroad to lie for the good of his country." Similarly, a surgeon general is an honest physician who goes to Washington to lie for his government. Elated by Satcher's manifesto, Michael M. Faenza, president of the National Mental Health Association, gushed: "This is a historic day. It's wonderful that we have a Surgeon General talking about mental health and mental illness, in a voice that has not been used in Washington before."[115] The fact that we hear this voice now is evidence that we have embraced pharmacracy, which promises to become the twenty-first century's grand utopian collusion between the state and the people.

CONCLUSIONS

Bodily diseases are physicochemical phenomena or processes *located in bodies*. Mental diseases are the names of unwanted personal habits or behaviors *located in social contexts*.

Psychiatry, like religion, is an institution for the regulation of human behavior—by rhetoric and repression, that is, by propaganda, persuasion, the threat of force, and the use of force. A person may abide by rules voluntarily or he may be compelled to do so by individuals or institutions authorized to use force. Medicine, especially psychiatry, now fulfills many of the existential and social functions previously fulfilled by religion.

Mind is not brain. Mental illness is not a true disease: it does not cause, explain or excuse criminal conduct; it is an attribute we attach to certain troubling, troublesome, and illegal behaviors. This conclusion does not rest on medical research; it rests on a refusal to be deceived. An eighteenth-century observer put it thus: "I know that a Triangle is not a Square, and that Body is not Mind, as the *Child knows that Nurse that feeds it is neither the Cat it plays with, nor the Blackmoor it is afraid of,* and the Child and I come by our Knowledge after the same Manner."[116]

6

PHILOSOPHICAL MEDICINE
Critique or Ratification?

Benevolence to the whole species, and want of feeling for every individual with whom the professors come in contact, form the character of the new philosophy.

Edmund Burke (1729–1797)[1]

A physician who is dependent only upon the usual guiding ethics—law, custom, and common sense—would not be able to defend the best interests of his patient when law, common practice, and conventional wisdom defined a patient's interests in terms that best serve society and not the individual.

Henry Greenberg* (1996)[2]

The health/disease question is irrelevant—we do not really have to know whether someone has a disease or not, and consequently we do not need a definition of "disease."

Germund Hesslow+ (1993)[3]

When I was a medical student, during World War II, philosophers were not concerned with medicine, physicians did not aspire to be philosophers,

*Henry Greenberg, M.D., is a distinguished cardiologist and clinical professor of medicine at Columbia University College of Physicians and Surgeons.
+Germund Hesslow has doctorates in both philosophy and physiology and is on the faculty of the University of Lund, Sweden.

bioethics was not a recognized medical or philosophical discipline, and there were no medical ethicists. Today, in the United States, there are some two hundred practicing "clinical ethicists."[4] One of them proclaims: "We are entering a truly new era of medicine, one in which philosophical, historical, and ethical reflection will no longer be viewed as alien and secondary, but rather as essential . . . paving the way for . . . a new, more humane medicine."[5] The opposite is more likely to be the case.

In the aftermath of World War II—stimulated partly by accounts of medical atrocities in Nazi Germany, partly by accounts of psychiatric atrocities in insane asylums at home, and partly by the medical-social problems associated with abortion and homosexuality—there suddenly emerged a new branch of academic inquiry, called "medical ethics." With great speed, medical ethicists established their own journals and proceeded to generate a vast literature, much of it devoted to justifying various medical interventions considered controversial. Almost overnight, medical ethics became a prestigious academic and medical discipline and a widely discussed topic in the popular press.

Most medical ethicists were, and are, philosophers, theologians, and physicians, a disproportionately large number of the latter being psychiatrists. The status of psychiatry as a medical specialty is marginal at best. Psychiatrists have a long history of violating basic human rights. Hence, the dominant role of psychiatrists in medical ethics casts a moral shadow over the field. The ethics of medical ethics is further jeopardized by the fact that much of the work is done by agents of the government or by professionals whose careers depend on grants from government agencies, often the National Institute of Mental Health (NIMH). The influence of that government agency on medical ethics and psychiatry has not received the attention it deserves. The very existence of the NIMH implies that mental diseases exist. Or, to use a different analogy, as the existence of the Vatican is premised on the legitimacy of theological authority, so the existence of the NIMH is premised on the legitimacy of psychiatric authority. This situation has virtually precluded unbiased philosophical inquiry into the ethics of psychiatry and has contaminated all of medical ethics.[6]

THE PHILOSOPHY OF MEDICINE: CRITIQUE OR RATIFICATION?

Philosophy—literally, the love of wisdom—is concerned with the theory of knowledge and with ethics. When we speak of the philosophy of a particular academic discipline or science—for example, the philosophy of history or philosophy of physics—we refer to a critical inquiry into the principles and values that determine what counts as knowledge in the field. Typical philosophical inquiries into prevailing mores, such as those of Socrates, have been *critiques* of the conventional views held by powerful authorities. Typical philosophical inquiries into prevailing medical and psychiatric practices are the opposite. For the most part, they are *ratifications* of conventional opinions, promoted by powerful medical, psychiatric, and political authorities.

The role of institutionalized "ethics" as an instrument for ratifying coercion as care is especially important in psychiatric ethics, many authorities in the field appealing to their own or to society's "moral intuition" as a guide to professional conduct. We must do better than this. National Socialist and Communist medical practices were considered ethical by Nazi and Soviet ethicists. Those examples ought to have taught us that one man's moral intuition is another man's crimes against humanity. Most of the ethical problems of modern medicine are rooted in the alliance between medicine and state, giving the physician power not only over the patient but also to shape cultural opinion and law. Hence, a medical ethicist worthy of the name must, following Socrates' example, be critical of medical power. He is not needed as yet another authority to undermine the citizen's privacy, dignity, and liberty.

Because the practicing physician must often balance a host of potentially conflicting interests—typically those of the patient against the needs of the patient's family or employer, the customs and laws of the country, and the physician's own personal needs—the ethical medical ethicist ought to be forthright about his own moral and political values and not conceal his views and recommendations with euphemistic phrases, such as "beneficence" or "the best interests of the patient." Those slogans may be used to rationalize virtually any medical intervention. Medical ethics itself requires unceasing ethical scrutiny.

The Ontology of Disease

Webster's defines ontology as "the science or study of being; . . . a theory concerning the kinds of entities and specifically the kinds of abstract entities that are to be admitted to a language." From the point of view of the pathologist, there is, as we saw, nothing abstract about what counts as a disease. A cirrhotic (sick) liver is obviously different from a normal (healthy) liver, just as a flat ("sick") tire is obviously different from an inflated ("healthy") tire. At bottom, the concepts of disease and health are no more complicated than that.

"Scientific medicine," Virchow emphasized, "has as its object the discovery of changed conditions, characterizing the sick *body*. . . . Its foundation is thus physiology."[7] The fact that animals can have, or can be made to have, many of the same diseases that human beings have is the basis for the important field of experimental medicine. Scientists can produce certain diseases in animals and can administer various drugs to them to determine their safety and therapeutic efficacy. Before World War II, philosophers writing about disease appreciated the elementary distinctions between disease and nondisease. Writing in 1937, Mortimer J. Adler stated: "It is clear that in the strict meaning of 'disease' only the body can suffer lesions; the intellect as such cannot be diseased, though it can be affected by a diseased body. Abnormalities which are not strictly diseases are the results of habit formation, contrary to the *norms* of good conduct; in other words, vicious characters."[8] Today, this view is considered "outmoded" and the language in which Adler had cast it is excoriated as lacking in compassion.

Many medical philosophers deal with the problem of behavior as nondisease by simply ignoring the pathological concept of disease. "Animals do not have diseases," asserted Peter Sedgwick, an English professor of politics and philosopher of medicine. Having unburdened himself of that insight, he exclaimed incredulously, "Who has ever imagined that spiders or lizards can be sick or diseased?," [9] and answered: "The blight that strikes at corn or at potatoes is a *human invention*. . . . Animals do not have diseases either, prior to the presence of man in a meaningful relation with them. A tiger . . . may be infected by a germ, trodden by an elephant, scratched by another tiger, or subject to the aging process of its own cells. It does not present itself as being ill. . . . Outside the significance that man attaches to certain conditions, *there are no illnesses or diseases in nature*."[10]

Sedgwick failed to distinguish between having a disease and being a patient (the tiger "does not present itself as being ill"); declared, in classic solipsistic style, that material objects do not exist unless they are seen and named by human beings (*"there are no illnesses or diseases in nature"*); and maintained that *"all sickness is essentially deviancy* . . . mental illness can be conceptualized just as easily within the disease framework as physical maladies such as lumbago or TB."[11]

DECONSTRUCTING THE CONCEPT OF DISEASE

My critics are fond of asserting that I "deny the reality of mental illness." It's not that simple. The person who insists that a whale is not a fish does not deny its existence. Asserting that the whale is a mammal is not a denial of its existence, it is a way of classifying the animal that contradicts the beliefs or claims of those who think it is a fish. Although the whale looks like a fish, lives in water, and unsophisticated people think it is a fish—philosophers do not accept the claim that it is a fish. Many behaviors look like diseases, are called "mental diseases," and psychiatrists think they are diseases—and most philosophers accept the claim that they are diseases.

114

When I say that mental illness is not an illness I do not deny the reality of the behaviors to which the term points, or the existence of the people who exhibit them, the suffering the denominated patients may experience, or the problems they create for their families. I merely classify the phenomena people call "mental illnesses" differently than do those who think they are diseases. When a lesion can be demonstrated, physicians speak of bodily illnesses. When none can be demonstrated, perhaps because none exists, but when physicians and others nevertheless want to treat the problem as a disease, they speak of mental illnesses. The term "mental illness" is a semantic strategy for medicalizing economic, moral, personal, political, and social problems.

Feeling constrained by the pathological concept of disease, many philosophers argue that the Virchowian concept may apply to disease as defined by the physician, but does not always apply to illness as experienced by the patient. This may or may not be true, but is beside the point. Scientific concepts typically are not the same as lay concepts. For the chemist, water is molecules, each containing two atoms of hydrogen and one of oxygen. For the lay person, it is simply water, used as a drink and useful for putting out fires. Chemists and firemen do not try to reconcile the differences between the scientific and lay concepts of water. The pathologist's and the priest's concepts of death differ in similar ways; they do not try to reconcile the differences. Why, then, are philosophers of medicine so eager to reconcile the differences between the scientific and lay concepts of disease? The evidence suggests that they do so because, faced with supporting or opposing certain well-established medical policies, they choose to support them. This applies with special force to psychiatric policies whose legitimacy depends on fudging the differences between diseases and nondiseases. The more closely we scrutinize the philosophers' neglect of, indeed scorn for, the classic Virchowian concept of disease, the more apparent it becomes that their aim is to replace the empirical-descriptive, biological definition of disease with a political-strategic, social definition of it.[12] This then justifies medicalizing social controls, especially psychiatric coercions and excuses.

Distinguishing Disease from Illness

In his frequently cited essay "On the Distinction between Disease and Illness," Christopher Boorse, professor of philosophy at the University of Delaware, approvingly quotes psychiatrist Ian Gregory's assertion: "While professionals have a major voice in influencing the judgment of society, it is the collective judgment of the larger social group that determines whether its members are to be viewed as sick."[13] This is starting off on the wrong foot. The key concepts of science are defined by scientists, not by lay persons or society.

Concepts such as mass, element, and gene are defined by physicists, chemists, and biologists, not by the individual or collective opinion of nonscientists. The claim that the pathologist's definition of disease ought to have no more scientific standing than "the collective judgment of the larger social group" is plain silly. Since Boorse agrees that "it seems doubtful that on any construal mental illness will ever be, in the mental health movement's famous phrase, 'just like any other illness,' "[14] it is not clear what he is getting at. Nevertheless, Boorse's paper is regularly cited as *proof that mental illness is not a myth.*

Without mentioning Boorse's essay, Horacio Fabrega, Jr., professor of psychiatry at the University of Pittsburgh, writes: "We really need two ideas, namely, disease and illness. . . . 'Disease' refers to a negative (i.e. unwanted) discontinuity or deviation in the condition of a *person.*"[15] Notice that Fabrega's definition rules out the possibility of plants and animals having diseases. Indeed, according to Fabrega, disease is not a condition of the body at all, it is a condition of the person. "The idea of disease as 'illness,'" he continues, "may be used to signify purely behavioral changes. . . . *the idea of illness applies principally to human groups and operates in a socio-political framework.*"[16]

A few more examples suffice. Arthur Kleinman, professor of psychiatry at Harvard, proposes a radical divorce of illness from disease. "Disease," he declares, "is what practitioners have been trained to see through the theoretical lenses of their particular form of practice. . . . The practitioner reconfigures the patient's . . . illness or problems as narrow technical issues, disease problems."[17] The professional's concept is "reconfigured," that is, distorted. The patient's, by implication, is unreconfigured, that is, undistorted (by professional or class prejudice). Leon Eisenberg, also professor of psychiatry at Harvard, agrees: "To state it flatly, patients suffer 'illnesses'; physicians diagnose and treat 'diseases.' "[18] Seeking to legitimize mental diseases as genuine diseases, he declares: "When physicians dismiss illness because ascertainable 'disease' is absent, they fail to meet *their socially assigned responsibility. It is essential to reintegrate 'scientific' and 'social' concepts of disease and illness as a basis for a functional system of medical research and care.*"[19]

When a surgeon finds that his patient has no disease that can be remedied by surgical treatment, his medical-ethical duty is to send the patient back to the referring physician, not "to reintegrate 'scientific' and 'social' concepts of disease and illness." When hematologists, ophthalmologists, and other nonpsychiatric physicians examine a patient and find no "ascertainable 'disease,'" their duty is to so inform the patient, not "to reintegrate 'scientific' and 'social' concepts of disease and illness." If psychiatry is a medical specialty, why should the psychiatrist's duty be different? The answer is clear: In the absence of objective measures for mental illness, the notion of finding evidence of "ascertainable mental illness" is devoid of meaning.

PHILOSOPHERS OF MEDICINE

Freud claimed that the aim of psychoanalysis was to make conscious in the patient or, better, in society, what was unconscious. He accomplished the opposite. He made unconscious what was conscious, transforming an honest quest for self-understanding into a corrupt pilgrimage for self-obfuscation.[20] I am afraid the same charge may be leveled against many medical philosophers. Instead of throwing light on disease and medicine, they cast shadows to conceal moral problems and political agendas.

K. W. M. Fulford: *Moral Theory and Medical Practice*

One of the most prestigious contributors to the literature of medical philosophy is K. W. M. Fulford, a professor at Oxford University. His book, titled *Moral Theory and Medical Practice,* has little to do with moral theory and even less with medical practice. Acknowledging that his aim is to give different meanings to the terms "disease" and "illness," Fulford maintains that mental illnesses are the same kinds of diseases as bodily illnesses and defends traditional psychiatric principles and practices. He proposes the following definition of disease: "First, the idea that 'illness' is a value term will be adopted as an assumption; next, *a hypothesis about 'disease' will be derived from this assumption.*"[21] Neither the pathologist in the laboratory, nor the clinician at the bedside, nor the suffering patient views disease as a *hypothesis derived from an assumption.* The utility of Fulford's interpretation clearly lies elsewhere.

"Contrary to the conventional view," Fulford continues, *"it is 'mental illness' rather than 'bodily illness' which is most like 'illness.* . . .' 'Mental illness' reveals, whereas 'bodily illness' conceals, not only the evaluative nature of 'illness' but also its logical origins in 'action.' "[22] When a veterinarian diagnoses a sick animal, he does not do so from "its logical origins in 'action,'" whatever that means. Clearly, Fulford's concept of disease has nothing to do with the accepted medical definition of the term. The following comment illustrates that his aim is to legitimize the psychiatric enterprise: "DSM-III and its successor DSM-R represent major advances in the classification of psychiatric disorders. . . . The success of these classifications is a direct result of the adoption of a descriptive approach to the definition of mental disorders, more or less consciously *emulating* the scientific basis of disease classification in physical medicine."[23] If mental illnesses are physical diseases, why is there a need to *emulate* "the scientific basis of disease classification in physical medicine?" The need to emulate is *prima facie* evidence that mental illnesses are not diseases. Nevertheless, Fulford maintains: "Once 'illness' and 'disease' are clearly distinguished, however, it becomes possible to compare like with like, 'mental illness' with 'physical illness,' 'mental disease' with 'physical disease.' . . . Physical illnesses are like mental illnesses in being constituted typically by mental, rather than physical, phenomena. . . . Our objective, here, is simply to mark the qualitative similarities between 'mental illness' and 'bodily illness.' "[24]

Ironically, this sort of philosophizing is now widely accepted as a daring advance over the so-called mind-body dualism. It is nothing of the sort. It is a regression to the concept of disease held in prescientific times or by people today who have no concept of scientific medicine, such as the Hmong, for whom "psychological problems do not exist . . . because they do not distinguish between psychological illness and physical illness."[25]

The practical import of Fulford's medical philosophy may be inferred from his views concerning problematic human situations. Throughout the book, Fulford defends, indeed lauds, psychiatric coercions, on what he regards as philosophical grounds. Citing the case of a suicidal bank manager hospitalized against his will, he writes: "This case, which is a clinically standard one, shows just how compelling is the moral intuition under which most compulsory treatment is carried out. Although it involves a clear infringement of liberty, few would disagree with the psychiatrist that he had 'no option' but to proceed as he did. Indeed, he might well have been judged negligent had he not done so."[26] In other words, the doctor was merely "following orders," to be sure not those of the national socialist state but those of the therapeutic state. Fulford recognizes that the psychiatrist is under legal duress to engage in the practice of coercive suicide prevention, a practice whose moral nobility and prudential validity he never questions. His account is a psychiatric justification, not a philosophical analysis, of the moral and political grounds for depriving innocent persons of liberty under psychiatric auspices. Phrases such as "moral intuition" and "few would disagree" are poor substitutes for moral reasoning.

Suppose that suicide were not considered a disease, would it still be morally justified to deprive people of liberty because they want to kill themselves? Would it be reasonable to entrust the job to psychiatrists and justifiable to call such preventive detention "medical treatment?"[27] Fulford fails to consider the arguments against viewing suicide as a disease or against coercive psychiatric suicide prevention. He is in good company. Mary Warnock, a distinguished British philosopher, endorses Fulford's defense of the special moral status of mental illness and the conventional moral justification for psychiatric coercion. In a "Philosophical Foreword" to *Moral Theory and Medical Practice*, she writes: "Dr. Fulford defends the concept of mental illness; and he argues convincingly that there can be theoretically sound moral justification for committing the mentally ill to hospital against their wishes . . . because the patient suffering from a psychotic illness has a *disrupted set of reasons* for his actions that it may be necessary, and justifiable, to commit him to hospital against his will."[28] Many people have reasons for their actions that others consider "disrupted," for example, Christian Scientists who reject medical treatment. Does Warnock believe that one person's opinion that another has a "disrupted set of reasons" for his actions is sufficient grounds for concluding that the other has a disease? And that such a diagnosis, per se, is adequate moral and political justification for depriving a person of liberty? Or is she simply supporting prevailing social policy, as did Cardinal Bellarmine in his famous confrontation with Galileo?

The difficulty with many philosophical analyses of medical practices may be that the commentators are ignorant of elementary medical concepts and facts. "A patient may have a disease, such as diabetes," writes Warnock, "but, if his disease is controlled, he may not be ill."[29] If Warnock means that the patient may not *feel ill*, she is right. However, since there is no cure for diabetes, the patient has the disease regardless of whether he feels its effects or is undergoing treatment for it. In the case of mental disease, the physician's statement forms the basis for concluding that the patient has a disease.

"The notion of 'dysfunction,'" Warnock continues, "belongs with disease."[30] This is wrong. The notion of dysfunction belongs with symptom and disability. Many diseases are asymptomatic and nondisabling (at least for a period of time). "To 'illness' on the other hand belongs the more complicated notion of a failure of action. A patient is ill if he cannot do certain things he ordinarily can do. His intentions and plans are disrupted, and he is aware of this whatever he and his doctor may know about the dysfunctioning of his body."[31] Assertions this absurd betoken what used to be called "invincible ignorance." A traveler stranded at an airport because his flight is canceled meets the criteria of having his intentions and plans disrupted, and "he is aware of this whatever he and his doctor may know about the dysfunctioning of his body."

My purpose here is not so much to present an extended critique of Fulford's or Warnock's views on mental illness as to show that their agenda is to negate the scientific concept of disease and instead define disease in a way that is completely independent of, and is unrelated to, somatic pathology.

Princeton philosopher Robert L. Woolfolk's concept of mental illness is similar to Fulford's (whose work he does not mention): "A malfunction/modularity-based model, no matter what definition of function we employ, allows us to place mental and somatic disorders on the same conceptual footing. . . . A mental organ, module, or device can malfunction, just as a bodily organ can; we only need be able to give it a scientifically acceptable characterization and attribute a function to it. Contemporary cognitive science approaches psychopathology in just this fashion."[32] A "mental organ, module, or device" is, of course, a metaphorical organ, module, or device.

I believe it behooves philosophers who write about mental illness to consider the actual uses to which nonphilosophers, who employ the concept in real life, put it.

Charles M. Culver and Bernard Gert: *Philosophy in Medicine*

Philosophy in Medicine, by Charles M. Culver and Bernard Gert, both at Dartmouth College, represents the most ambitious job of deconstructing disease so that nothing is left but its identity with mental illness. Although the thrust of their thesis is that mental illness is a *bona fide* disease and that psychiatry is an integral part of medicine, the book's subtitle, *Conceptual and Ethical Issues in Medicine and Psychiatry,* belies this view. If psychiatry were a part of medicine, it would be redundant to speak of "medicine *and* psychiatry."

Culver and Gert begin by asking: "Is alcoholism a disease? Are there any mental illnesses? Can there be rational suicide?" They continue: "For example, when Thomas Szasz asserts that mental illness is a myth, he is not simply making an empirical claim that can be conclusively verified or falsified by the collection of new information."[33] After briefly summarizing my views, they conclude: "It should be clear that this dispute cannot be settled solely by reference to the facts. What is needed is an analysis of the concept of illness. It may seem odd, but there have been few serious attempts to do this in the history of medicine until quite recently."[34] This is not true, unless one is prepared, as Culver and Gert are, to dismiss the Virchowian concept of disease. Indeed, the index to their book has no entry for autopsy, histology, lesion, or pathology.

Culver and Gert cite the definition of disease from a textbook of pathology as "any disturbance of the structure or function of the body or any of its parts," and dismiss it with this frivolous comment: "According to [this] definition, clipping nails and puberty are diseases . . . and [also] being tied to a chair."[35] Although the authors state that their "book is intended to demonstrate the value of philosophy in medicine,"[36] most of it is a defense of prevailing psychiatric ideas, institutions, and interventions, especially involuntary mental hospitalization and coercive suicide prevention. To accomplish this end, they, too, redefine disease, as follows: "*A person has a malady if and only if he has a condition, other than his rational beliefs and desires, such that he is suffering, or at increased risk of suffering, an evil (death, pain, disability, loss of freedom or opportunity, or loss of pleasure) in the absence of a distinct sustaining cause.*"[37] Note that the authors' definition of disease is detached from any connection with, or reference to, the body. If that is what disease is, why are medical students taught anatomy, pathology, and physiology? Culver and Gert support their definition of disease by citing George Engel's claim "that grief is a disease because it has the same characteristics as other diseases: ' . . . it involves suffering and an impairment of the capacity to function. . . . We can identify a constant etiological factor, namely, real, threatened, or *fantasied* object loss.' "[38] Here we encounter the familiar symptoms of medical imperialism: detaching the concept of disease from somatic pathology; changing the fundamental criterion for disease from lesion to cause, and treating fantasies as the causes and cures of *bona fide* diseases—in short, psychiatrizing disease.

Culver and Gert conclude: "We believe that the same criteria apply to mental conditions as to physical conditions. . . . Thus we differ from those who hold that mental illness either does not exist at all or else belongs in some fundamentally different category from physical illness. . . . there is no fundamental difference in kind between physical and mental maladies. *Both are defined by the suffering of evils.*"[39] The phrase "the suffering of evils" makes one think of innocent people in Nazi concentration camps and the Soviet Gulag, suffering because of the deeds of evil politicians. If suffering evils is regarded as a medical problem, then politics, religion, and life itself are swallowed up by medicine. That, indeed, seems to be Culver's and Gert's purpose when they philosophize about illness: "Our definition makes no distinction between physical and mental harms because we believe that, in defining maladies, both should be included. . . . To require someone suffering psychological harms that an alteration of physical functioning be present before her mental condition is labeled a malady seems ad hoc and unjustifiable. To illustrate that altered bodily processes are *not necessary to establish the existence of a malady, consider the case of schizophrenia.*"[40] Culver and Gert seem unconcerned that most psychiatrists believe that schizophrenia is a brain disease. They also believe that faking disease is a disease. "Munchausen patients [Munchausen syndrome is a type of malingering]," they explain, "differ from malingerers in that their symptom production and presentation, though often intentional, is unvoluntary [sic]."[41] "Culver and Gert's neologism, "unvoluntary," is an oxymoron—an action that is simultaneously intentional and involuntary (unvoluntary). Following psychiatric tradition, they justify psychiatric deprivations of liberty by asserting: "Most detentions are paternalistic acts. . . . They are done with the belief that they are for the patient's benefit."[42] It seems to me that authors who claim to present a philosophical justification for *medical practices that require the use of force* owe it to the reader to explain why psychiatrists, and only psychiatrists, should have the legal authority and professional duty to engage in such professionally rationalized violence. Priests and lawyers have no similar rights and duties to imprison their allegedly dangerous parishioners and clients.

Philosophers of Medicine and the Problem of "Real Disease"

Most medical philosophers are satisfied with falling back on the standard rationalizations of psychiatry. For example, Richard Hare, an emeritus professor at the University of Oxford, opines: "A psychiatrist may justifiably confine people for their own good (for example, to prevent suicide). It is the case that *in general* people who kill themselves are not acting in their own best interests."[43] Hare ignores that empirical studies of coercive psychiatric suicide prevention show that they promote rather than prevent suicide and that, ostensibly in the cause of preventing suicide, psychiatrists regularly violate their patients' rights.[44]

"The longer-term predictions of [patient] behavior . . . have been shown to be so inaccurate that the official policy of the American Psychiatric Association is that psychiatrists are incapable of making them," writes Robert Miller, professor of psychiatry at the University of Wisconsin.[45] He adds: "Clinicians who wish to secure hospitalization for patients who are perceived to need it clinically, but who decline to accept it voluntarily, *must make allegations of future dangerousness in order to obtain authority to provide the needed treatment.* . . . Predictions of dangerousness are rarely challenged in commitment hearings."[46]

Nevertheless, some prestigious philosophers go so far as to brand criticism of the concept of mental illness and objection to psychiatric coercion as an exercise in "antiscience." In an essay titled "The Growth of Antiscience," Paul Kurtz, an emeritus professor of philosophy at SUNY in Buffalo, states: "The most vitriolic attacks on science in recent decades have questioned its benefits to society." He lists ten types of such attacks, among them "opposition to psychiatry. . . . Thomas Szasz has no doubt played a key role here. . . . Many, like Szasz, even deny that there are mental illnesses, though there seems to be considerable evidence that some patients do suffer behavioral disorders and exhibit symptoms that can be alleviated by anti-psychotic drugs."[47] Note that Kurtz, a distinguished civil libertarian, fails to distinguish between voluntary and involuntary psychiatric interventions and invokes the authority of psychiatry and the alleged efficacy of forcible psychiatric drugging to justify depriving innocent people of liberty.

Because historians of medicine deal with interpretations of disease, they must have criteria by which to decide what counts as a disease; hence they cannot avoid being philosophers of medicine. What we find is that historians of medicine accept as disease whatever physicians call "disease"; at the same time, many of them recognize that mental illnesses are unlike bodily illnesses, but cannot bring themselves to declare mental illnesses to be nondiseases. English medical historian Roy Porter's essay on hysteria is illustrative. He writes: "For Szasz, hysteria is not a real disease, whose nature has been progressively cracked, but a myth forged by psychiatry for its own greater glory. Freud did not discover its secret; he manufactured its mythology. . . . Properly speaking, contends Szasz, *hysteria is not a disease* with origins to be excavated, but a behavior with meanings to be decoded. . . . Sidestepping mind-body dualisms,

Szasz thus recasts hysteria as a social performance, presenting problems of conduct, communication, and context."[48] Although Porter accurately summarizes my view that mental illnesses are not diseases (when I wrote *The Myth of Mental Illness*, hysteria was considered the paradigmatic mental illness, a role now played by schizophrenia), he fails to acknowledge its legal and social implications and disparages it by calling me "at bottom an old-school medical materialist [for whom] disease is really disease only if it is organic."[49] That is true but, in my view, it is not something to be ashamed of because it is anachronistic or naive.

Inasmuch as Fulford, Culver, Gert, Kurtz, and many other philosophers and psychiatrists direct much of their argument against my views, I cite, as a kind of rebuttal, the remarks of English social critic Robert Dixon: "*'Locking people up,' says Thomas Szasz, 'is a pivotal political act.'* . . . *Szasz observes that our laws on mental illness not only imprison without trial people innocent of any crime, they also pardon some who are found guilty in court.* . . . *Mind is confused with matter if we treat moral and ideological acts as if they were 'proven organic lesions,' argues Szasz* . . . *[and he] vividly describes how we apply a medical metaphor to what is actually a matter of manners, morals, politics, and justice. Szasz* . . . *unmasks a great absurdity, but has to watch the tide of opinion run the other way.*"[50]

Physicians and journalists are medical doctors and popularizers of science, not poets or humorists. Thus, when they call one or another distressing aspect of the human condition a disease, they must be taken seriously, the more so because they never suggest that they are using medical terms metaphorically. The following is a typical example: "Despite the great advances made in medicine, loneliness is the number one disease in the world today." This piece of foolishness comes from the pen of Kennedy Shortridge, professor of microbiology at the University of Hong Kong, and appeared in the prestigious medical journal *The Lancet*.[51]

Medical ethicists and medical philosophers have two choices. They can object to the expert's monopoly over the definition of mental disease or they can challenge his authority to use diagnoses as legal-political tools for incarcerating the innocent (civil commitment) and excusing the guilty (insanity defense). Without exception, medical ethicists and medical philosophers have chosen the first option. They favor "liberalizing" the concept of disease, in effect inflating it, recognizing all manner of competing definitions of illness, especially mental illness. Furthermore, they support retaining conventional psychiatric coercions and excuses. This is the path of progressive medicalization, subversion of the integrity of medical science, and loss of liberty through pharmacracy.

The second option, which I favor, is retaining the expert's privilege to define concepts pertaining to his expertise, in effect limiting the concept of disease to somatic pathology; and opposing *all psychiatric coercions and excuses*. This is the path of restoring free will and responsibility to individuals for their *behavior*, preserving the integrity of medical science, and protecting individual liberty and dignity from pharmacracy. The power to define scientific terms belongs to science. The power to use force belongs to the state. The twain shall never meet.

Relativizing the Concept of Disease

The tendency to expand the concept of disease by incorporating all manner of human problems into it has been accompanied by a corruption of the language of medicine and a disrespect for the precision of scientific discourse. Alongside the politically motivated *medicalization of nondiseases*, we witness the politically motivated *demedicalization of real diseases*.

In 1999, Glenn William Geelhoed, professor of surgery at George Washington University, reported the results of the mass treatment with depot injections of iodine of endemic hypothyroidism in a group of primitive people in the Congo. The treatment cured the disease, increased the people's energy level and fertility, and quickly led to unsupported population growth, destruction of the environment, and starvation.[52] Geelhoed's work generated considerable controversy, which he countered by asserting that "if one of our goals in health care is to go where the need is greatest," then the successful mass treatment of sick Africans was justifiable, indeed meritorious.[53] On its face, Geelhoed's argument is valid. However, it sidesteps several important issues: Did the recipients of his medical treatment perceive a problem? Did they seek relief from it? Were they willing to exchange something of value for what they presumably wanted and were given? What was their understanding of the consequences of the medical service they were getting? The answers to these questions are not clear.

Geelhoed's study demonstrated the obvious, but often neglected, differences between private health and public health. In the West, public health measures, such as programs aimed at lowering blood pressure, make people healthier as a group, but may not help any particular individual. Geelhoed's public health measure made individual patients healthier but harmed the group, by disrupting its adaptation to the environment. Like foreign aid projects that leave recipients collectively worse off than they were before, Geelhoed's medical aid may be criticized on moral and prudential grounds: he failed to consider whether the recipients perceived a problem or understood the consequences of solving it. However, instead of criticizing the study on these grounds, Jeremy Sugarman, a medical ethicist at Duke University, objected to Geelhoed's medical ethnocentrism—that is to his treating a *real dis-*

ease as if it were a disease. He wrote: "I am unsettled by the presumption that *the anatomic and physiologic indices of a Western investigator were assumed to be normal in another culture.*"[54] Is Sugarman also unsettled by such Western presumptions as the view that mosquitoes carry the parasites that cause malaria, even if African patients attribute having malaria to other causes?

The most important lesson we ought to draw from Geelhoed's study is that the presence of real disease does not automatically imply a need for treatment. However, since this lesson undermines the incessant search for diseases to explain human problems, Geelhoed's critics avoided making this point, preferring, in effect, to demedicalize hypothyroidism. The subtext of the controversy generated by Geelhoed's work is a complex set of motives, such as the zeal for "beneficence," one of the code words of contemporary medical ethics; subservience to powerful health care bureaucracies, such as the NIH and the WHO; and a misguided respect for the erroneous beliefs of so-called less-developed people. The controversy illustrates how medical ethics and medical politics have contaminated scientific medicine by relativizing its core concept, disease. Serious American medical scientists now seem to believe that hypothyroidism in Africans is not a disease, but social phobia in Americans is a disease.

CONCLUSIONS

Most philosophers of medicine do not understand or do not value the scientific and political significance of the core concept of disease as somatic pathology and ratify rather than critique problematic medical, especially psychiatric, practices. The result is that they oppose limiting the scope of the concept of disease to scientifically verifiable entities, support the claim that mental diseases are true illnesses, and defend traditional psychiatric coercions and excuses. Gone are critics such as C. S. Lewis. In 1953, he warned: "Of all the tyrannies a tyranny sincerely exercised for the good of the victims may be the most oppressive. . . . To be 'cured' against one's will and cured of states which we may not even regard as disease is to be put on a level with those who have not yet reached the age of reason or those who never will; to be classed with infants, imbeciles, and domestic animals."[55]

It is bad enough that our concept of disease is inflated and relativized; what is even worse is that it is *politicized and yet accepted as a medical standard.* Steven Hyman, M. D., director of the National Institute of Mental Health, declares: "More than 19 million Americans suffer from depression. . . . More than 2 million Americans have schizophrenia. . . . These illnesses . . . are real illnesses of a real organ—the brain. Just like coronary artery disease is a disease of a real organ—the heart."[56] Respected columnists repeat this canard as if it were a kind of higher truth the ignorant public refuses to heed. "Mental-health care is health care too," declares Anna Quindlen, "and mental illness is an illness. . . . Insurance providers should act like it. Hospitals and schools should act like it. Above all, we parents should act like it. Then maybe the kids will believe it."[57] It doesn't seem to occur to Quindlen that the experts on whose opinions she relies are the authorities that, in Lord Acton's words, "have worked for ages to build up the vast tradition of conventional mendacity."[58]

Physicians, philosophers, politicians, and pundits protest too much. The power to define disease belongs to, and is the responsibility of, medical scientists. The power to accept or reject medical treatment belongs to, and is the responsibility of, patients. The power to control criminals belongs to, and is the responsibility of, lawmakers, judges, and prison wardens. And the power to protect people's liberties belongs to, and is the responsibility of, the people.

7

POLITICAL MEDICINE
The Therapeutic State

Of all the enemies to public liberty, war is, perhaps, the most to be dreaded, because it comprises and develops the germ of every other. War is the parent of armies: from these proceed debts and taxes; and armies, and debts, and taxes are the known instruments for bringing the many under the domination of the few. . . . No nation could preserve its freedom in the midst of continual warfare.

James Madison (1795)[1]

War is the health of the State. It automatically sets in motion throughout society those forces for uniformity, for passionate cooperation with the Government in coercing into obedience the minority groups and individuals which lack the larger herd sense.

Randolph Bourne (1886–1918)[2]

The General Assembly hereby finds, determines, and declares that obesity is a serious medical problem. . . . Obesity ranks second only to smoking as a preventable cause of death. . . . The State Department shall classify obesity as a disease.

Colorado Senate Bill No. 00–034 (February 2000)[3]

One of the symbols of sovereign states is the postage stamp. Traditionally, American stamps depicted a famous American or an important historical scene. In 1893, to increase revenues, the U.S. Postal Service began to issue commemorative stamps. The first stamps with health-related themes—for example, a stamp depicting children playing and smiling, commemorating the centennial of the American Dental Association—appeared in 1959. In 1999, the Postal Service unveiled two stamps emblematic of the escalation of America's wars on diseases. On one, the inscription recommended: "Prostate Cancer Awareness: Annual Checkups and Tests"; on the other, it exhorted: "Breast Cancer: Fund the Fight. Find a Cure."[4]

THE MEDICALIZATION OF POLITICS

Webster's Third New International Dictionary defines the state as "the political organization that has supreme civil authority and political power and serves as the basis of government." Instead of offering definitions of the state, political scientists prefer to identify its characteristic features, for example, that it possesses "organized police powers, defined spatial boundaries, or a formal judiciary," or that "there is a deep and abiding association between the state as a form of social organization and warfare as a political and economic policy."[5] I regard monopoly on the legitimate use of force as the quintessential characteristic of the modern state. In this chapter, I focus on the beliefs and values that justify the possession of such force and the aims it serves.

The need to justify the use of force seems instinctive. For the child, the parent's power to coerce—by word or deed, intimidation or punishment—appears justified by his superior wisdom and by the child's innate lawlessness and socially imposed duty to become domesticated. The combination of the natural authority of the superior, the natural nonconformity of the subordinate and his need to learn the rules of the game and adhere to them, and the supreme importance of the welfare of the group (family, society, nation), which rests on conformity to social convention, form the template for religious, political, and medical justifications of coercive domination. Three familiar ideologies of legitimation result: (1) theocracy (God's will); (2) democracy (consent of the governed); and (3) socialism (economic equality, "social justice"). In the early 1960s, I suggested that modern Western societies, especially the United States, are developing a fourth ideology of legitimation. "Although we may not know it," I wrote, "we have, in our day, witnessed the birth of the Therapeutic State."[6] Since then, in articles and books, I have described and documented the characteristic features of this polity, medical symbols playing the role formerly played by patriotic symbols, the rule of medical discretion and "therapy" replacing the rule of law and punishment.[7]

It is undeniable that the state is primarily an apparatus of coercion with a monopoly on the legitimate use of violence. "Government," warned George Washington, "is not reason; it is not eloquence. It is power. Like fire it is a dan-

gerous servant and a fearful master."[8] Hence, as the reach of the legitimate influence of this "fearful master" expands, the sphere of personal liberties
contracts. What, then, ought to belong to the state, and what to the individual?
The history of the West may in part be viewed as the history of the growth of
freedom, characterized by a lively debate about where to draw the line between
the state's duty to safeguard the interests of the community and its obligation
to protect individual liberty. Accustomed to hearing phrases such as "freedom
of religion," "freedom of speech," and "the free market," we recognize that
each refers to a set of activities free from interference by the coercive apparatus
of the state. Should we, similarly, possess "freedom to be sick," "freedom to
make ourselves sick," "freedom to treat ourselves," "freedom to access medical
care," and so forth?

To intelligently debate where to draw the line between the welfare of the
community and the health of the individual, we must be clear about the legal
distinction between public health and private health. Edward P. Richards and
Katharine C. Rathbun, a law professor and public health physician, respectively, explain: "Public health is not about making individuals healthy; it is
about keeping society healthy by preventing individuals from doing things
that endanger others."[9] This is why preserving and promoting public health
often require coercion, whereas preserving and promoting private health require liberty and responsibility. "Persuading people to wear seatbelts, treat
their hypertension, eat a healthy diet, and stop smoking," Richards and
Rathbun continue, "is personal health protection. Stopping drunk drivers,
treating tuberculosis, condemning bad meat, and making people stop smoking
where others are exposed to their smoke is public health. . . . *Public health
should be narrowly defined* in terms of controlling the spread of communicable
diseases in society."[10] Instead of confronting the differences and conflicts between public health and private health, politicians, physicians, and lay people
debate slogans, such as the right to health, patient's bill of rights, patient autonomy, war on drugs, and war on cancer.

Medical Ideology and the Total State

In the nineteenth century, scientific medicine was in its infancy: disease was
defined by pathologists; effective remedies were virtually nonexistent; the term
"treatment" meant medical care sought and paid for by the patient; and the
state showed little interest in the concept of therapy.

Today, scientific medicine is a robust adult: physicians routinely perform
near-miraculous cures; disease is often defined by politicians and their lack-
eys—led by surgeons general; the state shows intense interest in the concept of
disease; and the term "treatment," is often used in lieu of the term "coercion."

Fifty years ago, few Americans others than politicians and physicians knew there was a bureaucrat in America called the "Surgeon General." Today, he is America's Physician General, preaching ceaselessly from the bully pulpit—a symbol and symptom of pharmacracy and of the growing power of the therapeutic State. Dan E. Beauchamp, an emeritus professor at SUNY–Albany, hails the sudden prominence of the Surgeon General as a sign of the "democratization" of health policy. He writes: "The role that democratic discussion now plays in health policy is perhaps best illustrated by the radical redefinition of the role of the U.S. Surgeon General from head of a rather obscure commissioned officer corps of the Public Health Service to our leading national spokesman on public health issues."[11]

Virchow longed for a future in which the physician *qua* Platonic philosopher would serve as a guide to the politician-king. "What other science," he asked rhetorically, "is better suited *to propose laws* as the basis of social structure, in order to make effective those which are inherent in man himself?"[12] He suggested that "once medicine is established as anthropology . . . the physiologist and the practitioner will be counted among the elder statesmen who *support the social structure.*"[13] Virchow was politically naive: he thought the future doctor would be a solid scientist and a wise leader, instead of, as is the case, a bureaucratic toady ignorant of scientific medicine. Furthermore, if the physician's task is to support the social structure, his actual job may be to harm, not help, the person called "patient."

We know that the proposition that *medical practice* is a science cannot be true.[14] Nevertheless, the idea is superficially attractive, even plausible. To resolve human problems, all we need to do is define them as the symptoms of diseases and, *presto*, they become maladies remediable by medical measures.

Medicine and the Metaphor of War

The illnesses first understood and conquered by scientific medicine were the infectious diseases. Because the response of the immune system to pathogenic microorganisms is readily analogized to a nation resisting an invading army, the military or war metaphor has become congenial to thinking about illness and treatment. When we speak about microbes "attacking" the body, antibiotics as magic "bullets," doctors as "fighting" against diseases, and so forth, we use metaphors to convey the idea that the doctor is like the soldier who *protects the homeland from foreign invaders*. However, when we speak about the war on drugs or the war on mental illness, we use metaphors to convey the idea that the state is like a doctor when it uses doctors as soldiers to *protect people from themselves*. In one case, we speak about doctors helping patients to overcome *diseases*, in the other, about doctors preventing citizens from *doing what they want to do.*

In the case of infectious diseases—the microbe as alien-pathogen threatening the host (the patient's body)—the war metaphor helps us understand the mechanism of the disease and justifies the coercive segregation (quarantine) of contagious persons, animals, or materials. In the case of psychiatric diseases—the war metaphor casting the mental patient in the role of alien-pathogen threatening the host (society)—the metaphor prevents us from understanding the problem misidentified as a disease: it convinces the patient's family, society, and sometimes the patient himself that the mental patient *is* (like) a pathogen, justifying the coercive segregation of the subject as "dangerous to himself or others." Failure to understand the abuses of the military metaphor in medicine and psychiatry precludes perceiving medical coercion as a "problem."

Viewing the state as primarily an apparatus of coercion with a monopoly on the legitimate use of force does not commit one to denying that the state can do good as well as evil. Probably no individual or institution is exclusively inclined to do evil. Moreover, doing evil to some often benefits others. The paradigmatic organ of the state is the army, which Robert Heinlein aptly characterized as "a permanent organization for the destruction of life and property."[15] The fact that armies are deployed to rescue people and help guard property after natural disasters does not alter their primary role.

It took centuries of terrible wars before people began to recognize that because the *state is, par excellence,* an instrument of violence, while the *church ought to be, par excellence,* an instrument of nonviolence, the two should get a divorce or at least a legal separation. Medicine and the state ought also to get a divorce, with primary custody of the citizens (as potential patients) granted to themselves, medicine having visitation rights. However, we do not view the relationship between medicine and the state the same way as we view the relationship between church and state. The reason may be that the physical ill health of the individual, unlike his spiritual ill health, can *directly* affect the physical health of the group. This has justified certain public health measures as legitimate instruments of state coercion. However, this reasoning does not justify state coercion as a morally legitimate instrument for protecting people from themselves. What should be the role of the state with respect to protecting the individual from diseases that do not by themselves pose a threat to others?

- Should protecting one's health be the responsibility of the individual, just as it is his responsibility to feed and house himself and provide for his spiritual health?

- Should the state assume responsibility for providing "health care," as it used to assume responsibility for providing "religious care" (a responsibility it still assumes in many parts of the world, even in some societies where church and state are in principle separated, for example Germany and Switzerland)?

- Should the state assume responsibility for protecting the individual from himself if—in the opinion of medical (psychiatric) experts—he poses a danger to his own health and well-being?

In my view, the coercive apparatus of the state ought to be as separate from the professional treatment of medical ill health as it is from professional treatment of spiritual ill health. Such a separation of medicine and the state is necessary for the protection and promotion of individual liberty, responsibility, and dignity.

Because the state has a monopoly on the legitimate use of force, it is the only institution legally empowered to wage war (and punish crime). Although the Constitution reserves to Congress the ultimate authority to engage the nation in war, that restraint is no longer operative. Since the end of World War II, American governments have waged wars, abroad and at home, by bureaucratic regulations and executive orders. Some of these wars have been justified on essentially medical grounds, for example the invasion of Panama. Illustrative of how far the blending of the concept of disease with the concept of war has gone is the declaration by the President and the Secretary of State, in June 2000, that AIDS in Africa poses a problem to America's *national security.*[16]

Regardless of why the government sends military personnel to foreign countries and of whether those in command call the operation "peace keeping" or a "war on narcoterrorism," the deployment of such force is an act of war. The enemy may be literal, an invading soldier, or metaphorical, a crop or chemical. The Germans and Japanese in World War II were literal enemies. The people who cause unrest in Haiti or Somalia, the peasants who grow coca in Colombia, the "drug lords" in Mexico, and the substances the government bans are metaphorical enemies. We sow metaphors of war, and reap literal violence. The fight against polio, let us remember, was called the March of Dimes, not a "war against polio," and it entailed no participation, assuredly no use of force, by the government. This is the background against which we ought to view America's unending wars on diseases and drugs.

To understand our present dilemma, we must understand the growth of the American state, especially since the Roosevelt years.[17] This was the period during which the United States became a complex, bureaucratic, regulatory, welfare state, a condition brought about by means of the time-honored political tactic of declaring a (national) emergency, requiring that all of the state's "human resources" be mobilized. "Every collective revolution," warned Herbert

Hoover (1874–1964), "rides in on a Trojan horse of 'Emergency.' It was the tactic of Lenin, Hitler, and Mussolini. . . . This technique of creating emergency is the greatest achievement that demagoguery attains."[18] The infamous George Jacques Danton (1759–1794) declared: "Everything belongs to the fatherland when the fatherland is in danger."[19] Two years later the fatherland repossessed his head. To the executioner about to guillotine him, he said: "Show my head to the people."[20]

In *Crisis and Leviathan,* Robert Higgs expands on this theme. "Knowing how the government has grown," he observes, "requires an examination of what, exactly, the government does: the growth of government has resulted not so much from doing more to accomplish traditional governmental functions; rather, it has resulted largely from the government's taking on new functions, activities, and programs—some of them completely novel, others previously the responsibility of the private citizen."[21] Higgs's thesis is that government expansion has been nurtured by a succession of "crises" that the government proceeds to "fix." After the crisis subsides, the new government functions remain, heaping bureaucracies upon bureaucracies. Although Higgs does not list health emergencies among the crises he discusses, they belong on top of the list.

Despite the evidence I have presented, well-respected social analysts maintain that the power and scope of the state are dwindling. In *The Rise and Decline of the State*, Martin van Creveld, professor of history at Hebrew University in Jerusalem, writes: "The state, which since the middle of the seventeenth century has been the most important and most characteristic of all modern institutions, is in decline."[22] How does Creveld arrive at this conclusion? By emphasizing growing popular resistance to the cost of socialist-inspired welfare state measures and by ignoring the growing popularity of a medically rationalized therapeutic state. Although Creveld's book runs to 438 pages, he does not mention the war on drugs or the pervasive influence of psychiatric-social controls. Others celebrate the "retreat of the State."[23] I agree with economist Robert J. Samuelson's observation that the government is "getting bigger because, paradoxically, we think it's getting smaller."[24] That is just one of the results of the politicization of the medicine and of medicalization of politics.

PHARMACRACY IN AMERICA

From 1776 until 1914, when the first antinarcotic legislation was enacted, the *federal government* played no role in *civilian* medicine. Medical licensure as well as the funding and management of state mental hospitals were functions of the *state* governments. After World War II, the situation changed rapidly and radically: the establishing of the National Institutes of Health, the enactment of Medicare and Medicaid legislation, and the war on drugs soon made medical expenditures the largest component of the national budget, eclipsing defense. The following statistics illustrate the explosive growth of the therapeutic state since the end of World War II and especially since the early 1960s.

- In 1950, funding for the NIMH was less than $1 million; ten years later, it was $87 million; in 1992, it reached $1 billion.[25] In 1965, when Medicare and Medicaid were enacted, their cost was $65 billion; in 1993, it was nearly $939 billion.[26] Between 1969 and 1994, the national mental health budget increased from about $3 billion to $80 billion.[27] Between 1968 and 1983, the number of clinical psychologists tripled, from 12,000 to more than 40,000; the number of clinical social workers grew from 25,000 in 1970, to 80,000 in 1990; and membership in the American Psychological Association grew from fewer than 3,000 in 1970 to more than 120,000 in 1993.[28]

- Between 1960 and 1996, total "national health expenditures" rose about 2.5-fold, from 5.1 percent of the gross domestic product (GDP) to 13.6 percent, while "federal government expenditures" on health rose more than sixfold, from 3.3 percent of the GDP to 20.7 percent. In 1995, total health expenditure, as percent of the GDP, was 13.6 percent in the United States, 10.4 percent in Germany, 8.6 percent in Australia, and 6.9 percent in the United Kingdom. In per capita health expenditures, the United States led all other countries by even bigger margins. The figures were $3,633 for the United States., $2,134 for Germany, $1,741 for Australia, and $1,246 for the United Kingdom.[29]

- Perhaps the most striking statistic is that between 1960 (before Medicare and Medicaid) and 1998, public expenditure per capita on health care increased more than 100-fold, from $35 to $3,633.[30]

The growth of the state is dramatically, and unequivocally, illustrated by its cost to the taxpayer, that is, the federal budget. The following figures are in nominal dollars (1 billion = 1,000 million, 1 trillion = 1,000 billion). In fiscal 1941, before the United States entered World War II, the budget was $13.6 billion; today, the war on drugs alone costs $19 billion. In 1942, the budget more than doubled, to $35.1 billion, in 1943 it was $78.5 billion, but it did not reach $100 billion until 1962. In the next 36 years the budget increased about sixteenfold, to 1.65 trillion in 1998.[31] According to James Buchanan, "In the seven decades from 1900 to 1970, total government spending in real terms increased forty times over, attaining a share of one-third in national product."[32]

The explosive expansion of the government after the 1960s is attributable largely to adding *civilian medical care* to the functions of the state. This transformation of medicine has utterly distorted the relationship between the private and public realms in general, especially between private health and public health. What makes the explosive expansion of the therapeutic state especially alarming is the widespread belief that the government is niggardly with respect to health care, especially mental health care—a myth largely fueled by the fact that the number of persons housed in buildings called "state mental hospitals" has decreased since the 1960s. I have documented elsewhere that while it is true that fewer people now reside in state hospitals than did thirty years ago, it is an illusion to think that the scope and power of psychiatry have diminished. The number of persons cared for, one way or another, by the mental health system has steadily increased since the end of World War II, as have mental health expenditures.[33] Despite these facts, the author of a "Special Report" in the *American Bar Association Journal* declares: "No one disputes that government support for the treatment of mental illness has dropped to dangerously low levels."[34]

The Anatomy of Pharmacracy: Secret Censorship as Health Care

The United States is the only country explicitly founded on the principle that, in the inevitable contest between the private and public realms, the scope of the former should be wider than that of the latter. That is what made America, especially in the nineteenth century, the "land of the free." "There is a balance of power," writes Bruce D. Porter, "between the state and civil society. This internal balance of power demarcates the line between the public and the private—*if a thing is public, it is subject to state authority; if it is private, it is not.*"[35] Pharmacrats want to abolish the private realm altogether. "It is the private sphere that is problematic for public health,"[36] declares Dan E. Beauchamp, seemingly not realizing that the private sphere is none of the business of public health.

It is a truism that people have more liberty in proportion as more aspects of their lives are private. The American people invited the state to take over the management of their health, and are now surprised that they have less control not only over the health care they receive but also over other aspects of their lives. Nor is that the end of the mischief. The more tax monies are spent on health care, the more firmly entrenched becomes the idea in nearly everyone's mind that caring for people's health requires not individual self-control, but political control, that is, control by deception, seduction, and coercion. The state commands vast resources of misinformation (propaganda) and seduction (money and other economic rewards) and has a monopoly of force (the law).

Censoring information has long been a tool of totalitarian states, both religious and secular. Such states need not and do not justify the practice by claiming that it serves the best interests of individuals. However, the First Amendment, guaranteeing freedom of the press, prohibits the American government from indulging in the despot's passion to deceive people, in their own best interest. Not only has the American government violated this prohibition, it has done so in secret and, after the practice was exposed, it defended it as a valuable weapon in the war on drugs.

Thanks to the sleuthing of the Internet magazine *Salon*, in January 2000 we learned that, for the past three years, the government has been secretly censoring many of the major television shows. What made the practice possible was a law requiring broadcast networks "to match the amount of 'anti-drug' advertising bought by the federal government with an equal amount of 'anti-drug' public-service announcements"—and the policy that if the "drug-czar's office approves a TV program's anti-drug content, the show itself can be credited against the requirement, allowing the network to then substitute full-price advertising for public-service announcements."[37] The arrangement posed a temptation for TV executives to augment their revenues by cooperating with the offers of the antidrug censors. "Under the sway of the office of President Clinton's drug czar, Gen. Barry R. McCaffrey, many of the most popular shows have filled their episodes with anti-drug pitches. . . . McCaffrey never let on that his office had been turned into a full-blown script-review board."[38] After the scheme was exposed, McCaffrey offered no apologies: "We plead guilty to using every lawful means to save America's children," declared his spokesman."[39] President Clinton was equally self-righteous: "I think this guy [McCaffrey] is intense and passionate and committed and we've got way too many kids using drugs, still."[40] Richard D. Bonnette, President and Chief Executive of Partnership for a Drug-Free America, lauded the censors: "The major television networks should be applauded for working with the Office of National Drug Control policy to include anti-drug story-lines in television shows."[41]

The Vatican's *Index of Prohibited Books* was a public document that proudly proclaimed the Church's struggle against values it considered subversive. In contrast, the clandestine nature of the White House Office of National Drug Control Policy's tampering with TV scripts is evidence that those responsible for it knew full well that they were subverting America's values, and perhaps its laws as well.

Private Health versus Public Health: Protecting People from Themselves

In the case of illness, drawing the line between the private and public realms requires careful consideration of many issues. As a first approximation, we may say that we have a "right to be sick"—an aspect of the right to be let alone—provided our illness does not *directly* harm others. We have a "right" to be sick with hay fever, because it does not endanger others, but we do not have a right to be sick with infectious tuberculosis, because it endangers others.

Yet, even such a seemingly uncontroversial example as hay fever oversimplifies the matter. The person suffering from hay fever may ingest antihistamines to alleviate his symptoms that, in turn, may render him just as impaired to drive an automobile as would intoxication with alcohol. In fact, simply being a young adult or an old adult makes the person, statistically, a dangerous driver. What constitutes a danger to the public depends partly on what people perceive as a risk, a perception shaped by subjective judgment rather than statistical probability, and partly on whether people perceive a particular risk as under their own control or as not under their own control. Regardless of the statistical risk, people do not worry much about risks they believe they can control.

To complicate matters, the sickness of persons and the sickness of populations represent very different problems, for patients, physicians, and politicians. Private health measures that benefit the individual may help or harm the community. Public health measures that benefit the community may help or harm the individual. The potential conflict between private health and public health is an integral part of the tension between civil society and the state. In his paper "Sick Individuals and Sick Populations," epidemiologist Geoffrey Rose notes that "a preventive measure which brings much benefit to the population offers little to each participating individual. This has been the history of public health—of immunization, the wearing of seatbelts, and now the attempt to change various life-style characteristics. Of enormous potential importance to the population as a whole, these measures offer very little—particularly in the short term—to each individual."[42]

Dealing with health care as a public good raises certain questions, such as: Can we create an insurance system that makes every treatment, deemed useful or necessary by a physician, affordable by and available to every member of the community? How can we calculate the cost of health insurance if medical science and technology create, and people clamor for, ever more and more expensive treatments? If people take good care of their health and live longer, what cost do they impose on those who pay their pensions or other old-age benefits? If the community pays for the treatment of those who fall ill, doesn't it inevitably acquire a claim on its members to try as hard as they can not to fall ill? Doesn't the community also acquire an interest in identifying and penalizing those who frivolously neglect their health or make themselves deliberately ill?

If we assume that people truly value their health, why don't we expect them to be willing to spend at least as much on medical care as they do on drinking, smoking, gambling, entertainment, and veterinary care for their pets? If people do not value their own health, then it's a folly twice over for the taxpayer to pay for their health insurance. In other words, why don't we means-test for health care coverage funded by tax monies? And why don't we model health insurance on private casualty insurance with a *substantial deductibility clause*—the insured being responsible for his own health care up to, say, 10 percent of taxable income, before becoming eligible for reimbursement? Indeed, shouldn't we try to return to the situation where medical care was available mainly to those who were able and willing to pay for it, with care to those who could not being distributed on some other basis?

These are hard questions that most people and all politicians prefer to avoid. Instead, politicians pander to the public with slogans promising health-care benefits without health-care responsibilities, and people like it that way. However, with the increasing cost of health insurance and the mounting dissatisfaction by both patients and doctors of mandated "insurance" schemes for health-care coverage, we ought to confront rather than shirk these questions. The truth is that, in the days before the federal government went into the business of health care, poor people received free medical services, often of very good quality, at municipal and teaching hospitals. It is doubtful that they receive better care now, but those who can pay often receive worse care than they did formerly. (The terms "better" and "worse" refer here to the human, not the technical, quality of the service.) Moreover, physicians are far less proud of, or satisfied with, being physicians than they were fifty years ago.

The advocates of pharmacratic politics threaten liberty because they obscure or even deny the differences between the kinds of risks posed by a public water supply contaminated with cholera bacilli and the risks posed by a private life-style that includes the recreational use of a prohibited psychoactive drug. The individual cannot, *by an act of will*, provide himself with a safe public water supply, but he can, *by an act of will*, protect himself from the hazards of smoking marijuana. What makes coercive health measures justified is not so much that they protect everyone equally, but that they do so by means not available to the individual. By the same token what makes coercive health measures unjustified is not only that they do not protect everyone equally, but that they replace personally assumed self-protection by self-control with legal sanctions difficult or impossible to enforce. The rhetoric of categorizing certain groups—typically, children or the residents of neglected neighborhoods—as "at risk," needs to be mentioned here. The term implies that the persons in question lack self-control and hence need the help of the government to protect them from certain kinds of temptations. Health statists on both the left and right agree.

Gerald Dworkin, for example, believes that "a man may know the facts [about the dangers of smoking], wish to stop, but not have the requisite willpower. . . . In [such a case] there is no theoretical problem. We are not imposing a good on someone who rejects it. *We are simply using coercion to enable people to carry out their own goals.*"[43] This is coercive paternalism in pure culture. I maintain that the only means we possess for ascertaining that a man wants to stop smoking more than he wants to enjoy smoking is by observing whether he stops or continues to smoke. Moreover, it is irresponsible for moral theorists to ignore that coercive sanctions aimed at protecting people from themselves are not only unenforceable but create black markets and horrifying legal abuses.

The idea that it is the duty of the state to protect people from themselves is an integral part of the authoritarian, religious-paternalistic outlook on life—now favored by many atheists as well. Once people agree that they have identified the one true God, or good, it follows that they must guard members of the group, and nonmembers as well, from the temptation to worship false gods or goods. The post-Enlightenment version of this view arose from a secularization of God and the medicalization of good. Once people agree that they have identified the one true reason, it follows that they must guard against the temptation to worship unreason, that is, madness.

Confronted with the problem of "madness," Western individualism was ill prepared to defend the rights of the individual: modern man has no more right to be a madman than medieval man had a right to be a heretic. In the seventeenth century, when madness appeared in its modern guise, the problem it presented resembled not only the problem of heresy but also the problem of disease, especially of the brain. Madness was perceived as an illness of the mind, due to a hypothecated disease of the brain, an image that invited conflating risk to the public with risk to the self—hence the view of the insane person as "dangerous to himself and/or others." This verbal formula has justified involuntary mental hospitalization for centuries. There is a large body of literature on this subject, to which I have contributed my share. I shall say no more about it here. Instead, I shall limit the discussion to a few remarks about medical-legal coercions whose avowed aim is to protect *mentally healthy* people from themselves.

Aside from suicide, whose legal-political status is obscured by its being authoritatively attributed to mental illness, a classic contemporary example of potentially self-injurious behavior is riding a motorcycle without a helmet.[44] (That riding a motorcycle *with* a helmet is also dangerous is beside the point here.) How do courts interpret the constitutionality of prohibiting people from riding a motorcycle without a helmet? Can motorcycle helmet laws be justified by invoking the police power—inherent in the sovereignty of states, enabling the legislatures "to act for the protection of the public health, safety, morals, and general welfare"[45]—which, however, is silent about protecting people from themselves? Some authorities say yes, some say no; the answer depends on whether the observer regards the subject's behavior as a private matter that affects only him, or as a public matter that affects others as well. One court "held the statute to be an unconstitutional exercise of the police power," citing the legal maxims: "The individual is not accountable for his actions, insofar as these concern the interest of no person but himself" and "So use your own that you do not harm that of another."[46] Another court held that the state has an interest in having robust, healthy citizens and, therefore, "the statute forcing an individual to protect himself falls within the scope of the police power."[47]

The issue comes down to *whether the individual is viewed as a private person or as public property*: the former has no obligation to the community to be or stay healthy, the latter does. In proportion as medical care is provided by the state, doctors and patients alike cease to be private persons and forfeit their "rights" against the opposing interests of the state. Declares Alan I. Leshner, head of the National Institute of Drug Abuse (NIDA): "My belief is that today, in 1998, you [the physician] should be put in jail if you refuse to prescribe S.S.R.I.s [Selective Serotonin Reuptake Inhibitors, a type of so-called antidepressant medication] for depression. I also believe that five years from now you should be put in jail if you don't give crack addicts the medication we're working on now."[48] In plain English, Leshner dreams of *coercing physicians to forcibly drug patients.*

History teaches us that we ought to be cautious about embracing professional protectors as our guardians: they often demean, coerce, and injure their beneficiaries and do their best to render them abjectly dependent on their tormentors. Transforming the United States from a constitutional republic into a therapeutic state has shifted the internal balance of power in favor of the government and against the individual. Ironically, this shift was accompanied by widespread complaints by the cognoscenti about a surfeit of autonomy plaguing Americans.[49] They mistake for autonomy what is in fact selfishness engendered by the growth of pharmacratic regulations and the therapeutic state. (I use the term "pharmacratic regulations" to refer to controls exercised by bureaucratic health-care regulations, enforced by health-care personnel, such as alcohol treatment and other addiction programs, school psychology, suicide prevention, and the mandatory reporting of personal [mis]behavior as part of the duties of pediatricians, internists, psychiatrists, and other health-care personnel.)

COERCION AS TREATMENT: JUSTIFYING PHARMACRACY

Coercion masquerading as medical treatment is the bedrock of political medicine. Long before the Nazis rose to power, physician-eugenicists advocated killing certain ill or disabled persons as a form of treatment for both patient and society. What transforms coercion into therapy? Physicians *diagnosing* the subject's condition a "disease," *declaring* the intervention they impose on the victim a "treatment," and legislators and judges *ratifying these categorizations* as "diseases" and "treatments." Simply put, the pharmacrat's stock-in-trade is denying the differences between medical care sought by patients and imposed on them against their will—in short, defining violence as beneficence.

The normal applications of the criminal law tell us that the difference between depriving a person of his liberty and depriving him of his life is a matter of degree, not kind. The history of religious persecution teaches the same lesson, more dramatically. Medical ethicists and psychiatrists ignore this evidence: they embrace medicalized deprivation of liberty, provided it is called "hospitalization," "outpatient commitment," "drug treatment," and so forth. Many of them approve even deprivations of life, provided it is called "physician-assisted suicide" or "euthanasia." Let me restate the elements necessary to qualify a medical *intervention* as a medical *treatment*. From a scientific point of view, an intervention counts as treatment only if its aim is to remedy a true disease; the identity of the person doing the remedying does not matter: self-medication with an analgesic for pain, or with an antihistamine for hay fever, counts as treatment. From a legal point of view, an intervention counts as treatment only if it is performed by a physician licensed to practice medicine, with the consent of the subject or his guardian; disease, diagnosis, and medical benefit are irrelevant. Consensual treatment is treatment only if the patient has a true disease, regardless of whether it is effective or does more harm than good; nonconsensual "treatment" is assault, even if it cures the patient of his disease.

The Perversion of Medicine: Disease as "Treatability"

"When meditating over a disease," wrote Pasteur, "I never think of finding a remedy for it."[50] When the pharmacrat meditates over disease, he thinks of nothing but how to remedy it; and because he views benevolent coercion as treatment, he discovers diseases where his patient/victim sees only behaviors that the pharmacrat wants to change or punish.

The idea of defining disease in terms of treatability is not new. The prescientific physician and his clients often perceived illness this way. The principal difference between the old-fashioned quackery of, say, Mesmer, and the new-fangled quackery of, say, our surgeons general, is that Mesmeric "treatments" were never imposed on persons against their will, whereas the "treatments" endorsed by the surgeons general often are.

Nazi pharmacracy was based on the premise that the Jew was a cancer on the body politic of the Reich; it had to be removed at any cost. American pharmacracy is based on the premise that the individual with a dangerous disease, epitomized by the drug abuser, is a threat to the well-being of the nation; he has to be cured at any cost. In a brief article in *JAMA,* Leshner repeats this theme three times: "There are now extensive data showing that addiction is eminently treatable"; "addiction is a treatable disease"; "overall, treatment of addiction is as successful as treatment of other chronic diseases, such as diabetes, hypertension, and asthma."[51] Leshner studiously refrains from acknowledging that "treatment" for "addiction" is typically imposed on the subject by force.

Sally Satel, a psychiatrist at Yale University, is more forthright. "As a psychiatrist who treats addicts," she writes in an op-ed essay in the *Wall Street Journal*, "I have learned that legal sanctions—either imposed or threatened—may provide the leverage needed to keep them alive by keeping them in treatment. Voluntary help is often not enough."[52] The essay was titled "For Addicts, Force Is the Best Medicine." It does not bode well for liberty that the editors of even the *Wall Street Journal* apparently agree.

The proposition that the use of illegal drugs is a brain disease poses problems of its own. Brain diseases cannot be treated without the patient's consent. How, then, do Leshner, Satel, and others justify using force to treat *this* brain disease, but not others? Satel declares: "Addicts would be better off if more of them were arrested and forced to enroll in treatment programs . . . [this is] the essence of humane therapy."[53] The truth is that persons with real brain diseases need not be coerced into treatment because they can be persuaded to accept it. Is it any surprise that coercion is necessary to treat nondiseases?

In June 2000, Judith S. Kaye, chief judge of the State of New York, announced that "[New York] State courts will start using their 'coercive' powers immediately to get nonviolent drug offenders into treatment programs." Although defendants are under duress to accept "treatment," the therapists maintain that "accepting treatment is ultimately *voluntary*. . . . To be eligible, offenders will have to be . . . *willing to plead guilty*. . . . Even if a defendant chooses to stand trial, the judges and district attorneys will still have the discretion to refer them to drug treatment until trial. *If they are found not guilty, in all likelihood treatment will be continued,* said a court spokesman. . . . If they relapse, they will go to jail, most likely receiving stiffer sentences than normally given now."[54] This is an example of what happens to the concepts of disease, treatment, and voluntariness when politicians define illness and treatment.

Judge Kaye is proud of what she calls her "hands-on court" that promotes "problemsolving." The problem she has in mind is how to get people to stop doing what they like to do—in this case, using illegal drugs. What makes Judge Kaye think that the drug-treatment sentences she imposes solve drug problems? "We know," she writes, "that a defendant in a court-ordered drug treatment is twice as likely to complete the program as someone who gets help voluntarily."[55] The fact that drug prisoners complete court-ordered "programs" proves that they want to be free of meddling judges, not that they are free of the desire to take drugs. Moreover, completing a "drug treatment program" means simply being present at required meetings; it doesn't entail acquiring new knowledge or skills, as does completing an academic program. The result of Judge Kaye's sentence is exactly the opposite of what happens in a genuine educational program: It is unlikely that a person participating in such a program against his will would complete it, but it is likely a person who participates voluntarily (and pays for it) would do so.

Stories of judges practicing therapeutic jurisprudence abound in the media.[56] In Dade County, Florida, persons "caught using or purchasing drugs are considered 'clients' or 'members' rather than 'offenders' or 'defendants' . . . instead of trying to prosecute the defendant, the district attorney becomes part of the Drug Court team trying to help the defendant toward recovery."[57] A judge in Florida uses the phrase "*therapeutic jurisprudence' to describe the court's role as a facilitator of the healing process. . . . 'This is a helping court . . . which defendants enter voluntarily.'* "[58] Sadly, we have no Menckens or Orwells, warning people against Gulliverian tales of court-coerced habit retraining portrayed as "voluntary treatment" and courtrooms characterized as places that "defendants enter voluntarily."

Leading physicians fuel the propaganda for therapeutic coercions as remedies for social problems. In 1992, then Surgeon General C. Everett Koop and then editor in chief of *JAMA* George D. Lundberg declared: "One million US inhabitants die prematurely each year as a result of intentional homicide or suicide. . . . We believe violence in America to be a public health emergency."[59] Being murdered and dying voluntarily are here treated as similar phenomena and both are categorized as preventable diseases posing a "public health emergency." Articles about smoking, violence, and war are staples in the pages of *JAMA*. Some typical titles: "Tobacco Dependence Curriculum in US Undergraduate Medical Education."[60] "The Medical Costs of Gunshot Injuries in the United States."[61] "The Future of Firearm Violence Prevention."[62] "War and Health: From Solferino to Kosovo."[63] "What Can We Do about Violence?"[64]

In Britain, too, the medical establishment is solidifying its marriage to the state. In July 1999, the British Medical Association proposed that in order to increase "the number of donated organs, everyone should be assumed to be a donor unless they opted out."[65] With body ownership vested in the state, it is reasonable that the state should decide what counts as disease and treatment. In July 1999, a three-judge Court of Appeals panel in Britain ruled that the National Health Service (NHS) "wrongly regarded transsexualism as a state of mind that did not warrant medical treatment rather than as an illness. . . . [The judges ordered the NHS to] provide sex-change operations for transsexuals because they suffer from a *legitimate illness. . . .* About 1,000 transsexuals . . . will be entitled to the $13,000 sex-change surgery free of charge."[66] According to the judges, sex-change operation is *the proper treatment of a recognized illness."*[67] Recognized by whom? The bureaucrats of the therapeutic state.

In September 1999, the *Sunday Times* (London) reported that "the government is considering proposals to appoint secular 'vicars,' paid for by the state, to give pastoral care to families . . . offering pastoral advice and urging parents who do not attend church to put their children through a 'civil naming ceremony.' "[68] Evidently in vain did Daniel Defoe (1660–1731) warn: "Of all plagues with which mankind are cursd, / Ecclesiastic tyranny's the worst."[69] Secularism may protect us from the dangers of theological tyranny, but it does not protect us from the dangers of therapeutic tyranny. Electing a national leader by a majority of the people's votes may protect us from being ruled by an aristocracy, but it does not protect us from being ruled by a pharmacracy.

MEDICAL IDEOLOGY, PUBLIC HEALTH, AND SOCIALISM

Before considering the connections between Medicine and the state in National Socialist Germany, it may be instructive to briefly review the connections among antipoverty policies, public health measures, and the state.

Health, Poverty, and the State

For centuries, the relief of both poverty and illness, especially illness affecting the poor, was the responsibility of the church. "It is interesting to notice," wrote socialist dreamers Sidney and Beatrice Webb in 1910, "that the Public Health medical service and the Poor Law medical service sprang historically from the same source, namely the prevalence of disease among the pauper class, and the economy of diminishing it."[70] In the modern world, the state assumes both functions. Since World War II, the relief of illness has been increasingly perceived as a duty the state owes all its citizens.

The subvention of medical care by the state creates many problems, as we have seen already. Becoming ill and recovering from illness have a great deal to do with motivation, personal habits, and self-discipline. The Webbs, though ardent lovers of Leviathan, recognized this fact and warned against it, anticipating the criticisms of Ludwig von Mises, Leviathan's ardent enemy. "The very humanity and professional excellence of the Poor Law infirmary," the Webbs explained, "*constitute elements in the breaking down of personal character and integrity, and may even be said actually to subsidize licentiousness, feeble-mindedness, and disease."*[71] To prevent the cure from being worse than the disease, the Webbs proposed that "the curative treatment of individual patients by the Public Health Service . . . [be accompanied by] a *constant stream of moral suasion, and when necessary, disciplinary supervision*, to promote physical self-restraint and the due care of offspring."[72]

In the Soviet Union, the socialization of the economy led to widespread economic dissatisfaction. In Western democracies, the socialization of medicine is now leading to a similar widespread dissatisfaction with medicine, among patients and physicians alike. Since the interests of the state as producer of goods or provider of medical services are not the same as the interests of people as consumers or patients, this result is hardly surprisingly.

Health and the National Socialist State

Hitler recognized that the direct takeover of private property provokes powerful emotional and political resistance. One of the secrets of his rise to power was that he managed to portray the National Socialist movement as opposed to such a measure, indeed to Communism itself. As Robert Proctor notes, Hitler understood that there was no need to "nationalize industry when you can nationalize the people."[73] I want to emphasize here that I regard "right-wing" Nazism and "left-wing" Communism not as two antagonistic political systems, but as two similar types of socialism (statism)—one brown, or national, the other red, or international. Both kinds of statists were very successful in their efforts to undermine autonomy and destroy morality.

The therapeutic state as a type of total state with a sacred and therefore unopposable mission is not a new historical phenomenon. The theological state, the Soviet state, and the Nazi state may be viewed as former incarnations of it.[74] To illustrate and underscore the problems intrinsic to the alliance between modern medicine and the modern state, I shall briefly review the anatomy of National Socialist Germany as a type of therapeutic state.

From the beginning of his political career, Hitler couched his struggle against "enemies of the state" in medical rhetoric. In 1934, addressing the Reichstag, he boasted: "I gave the order . . . to burn out down to the raw flesh the ulcers of our internal well-poisoning."[75] National Socialist politicians and the entire German nation learned to speak and think in such terms. Werner Best, Reinhard Heydrich's deputy, declared that the task of the police was "to root out all symptoms of disease and germs of destruction that threatened the political health of the nation. . . . [In addition to Jews,] most [of the germs] were weak, unpopular and marginalized groups, such as gypsies, homosexuals, beggars, 'antisocials,' 'work-shy,' and 'habitual criminals.' "[76]

None of this was a Nazi invention. The use of medical metaphors to justify the exclusion and destruction of unwanted persons and groups antedates Hitler's rise to power and flourishes today. In 1895, a member of the Reichstag called Jews "cholera bacilli."[77] In 1967, Susan Sontag, the celebrated feminist-liberal writer, declared: "The truth is that Mozart, Pascal, Boolean algebra, Shakespeare, parliamentary government, baroque churches, Newton, the emancipation of women, Kant, Marx, Balanchine ballets, *et al.*, don't redeem what this particular civilization has wrought upon the world. *The white race is the cancer of human history*; it is the white race and it alone—its ideologies and inventions—which eradicates autonomous civilizations wherever it spreads, which has upset the ecological balance of the planet, which now threatens the very existence of life itself."[78]

Despite all the evidence, the political implications of the therapeutic character of Nazism, and of the use of medical metaphors in modern democracies, remain underappreciated or, more often, ignored. It is a touchy subject, not because the story makes psychiatrists in Nazi Germany look bad. That has been accepted and dismissed as an "abuse of psychiatry." Rather, it is a touchy subject because it highlights the dramatic similarities between pharmacratic controls in Germany under National Socialism and in the United States under what is euphemistically called the "free market."

Nazi Pharmacracy: I. Socialist Health Care

The definitive work on pharmacracy in Nazi Germany is *Health, Race and German Politics between National Unification and Nazism, 1870–1945*, by Paul Weindling, a scholar at the Wellcome Institute for the History of Medicine in London. Unlike many students of the Holocaust, Weindling does not shy away from noting the similarities between the medicalization of politics and the politicization of health in Nazi Germany and in the West. Many of Weindling's observations and comments about Nazi Germany as a therapeutic state (a term he does not use) sound as if they were addressed to conditions in the United States today. He writes:

- Scientifically-educated experts acquired a directing role as prescribers of social policies and personal lifestyle. . . . Science and medicine provided an alternative to party politics, by forming a basis for collective social policies to remedy social ills.[79]
- The sense of responsibility of the doctor to sick individuals weakened as awareness dawned of the economic costs of poverty and disease. . . . Medicine was transformed from a free profession . . . to the doctor carrying out duties of state officials in the interests not of the individual patient but of society and of future generations. . . . Doctors became a part of a growing state apparatus.[80]

Weindling retraces the political-economic history of modern medicine, reminding us that "in 1868 medicine was proclaimed a 'free trade,' open to all to practice ... without legal penalties against quackery. ... Leaders of the profession such as Rudolf Virchow were convinced that scientific excellence guaranteed the future of the profession."[81] *That* was a free market in medicine. Today, in contrast, trade in medical goods and services is stringently regulated by the state.

Long before Hitler rose to power, observes Weindling, physicians "sought to colonize new areas for medicine, such as sexuality, mental illness, and deviant social behavior. What had been private or moral spheres were subjugated to a hereditarian social pathology. ... As the medical categories invaded the terrain of social categories, the greater became the potential for creating a society corresponding to a total institution."[82] Deception and self-deception by medical rhetoric were popular as far back as 1914, when German military service was glorified "as healthier than urban life. The fresh air and exercise of the front meant that it could be a vast open air sanatorium. Another indicator of health was the fall in the number of mental patients and a decrease of suicides."[83] War, indeed, is the political health of the state and the mental health of the individual.

Bedazzled by the myth of mental illness and seduced by psychiatry's usefulness for disposing of unwanted persons, the modern mind recoils from confronting the irreconcilable conflict between the political ideals of a free society and the coercive practices of psychiatry. Let us keep in mind that psychiatry began as a statist enterprise: the insane asylum was a public institution, supported by the state and operated by employees of the state. The main impetus for converting private health into public health came, and continues to come, from psychiatrists.

In 1933, the year Hitler assumed power, a law was passed against "compulsive criminality . . . enabling preventive detention and castration . . . [for] schizophrenia, manic-depression, [etc.]. . . . The medical profession and especially psychiatrists benefited greatly from the drive for sterilization."[84] Reich Health Leader (*Reichgesundheistführer*) Leonardo Conti (1900–1945) stated that "no one had the right to regard health as a personal private matter, which could be disposed of according to individualistic preference. Therapy had to be administered in the interests of the race and society rather than of the sick individual."[85]

In 1939, medical killing in Germany went into high gear. "Reliable helpers were recruited from the ranks of psychiatrists," who defined lying for the state as a higher form of morality: "Each euthanasia institution had a registry office to issue the false [death] certificates."[86] In the case of tuberculosis, modern diagnostic technology was employed as a tool for determining who qualifies for therapeutic killing: "In occupied Poland and the Soviet Union, SS X-ray units sought out the tubercular, who were then shot. It is estimated that 100,000 died in this way."[87]

The more power physicians exercised, the more intoxicated with power they became. "The doctor was to be a Führer of the *Volk* to better personal and racial health. . . . Terms like 'euthanasia' and 'the incurable' were a euphemistic medicalized camouflage with connotations of relief of the individual suffering of the terminally ill."[88] During all the carnage, the Nazis remained obsessed with health: "A plantation for herbal medicines was established at the Dachau concentration camp."[89]

Nazi Pharmacracy: II. Waging War for Health

In *The Nazi War on Cancer*, Robert N. Proctor, professor of history at Pennsylvania State University, remarks on the similarities between pharmacratic controls in Nazi Germany and the United States today, only to dismiss them as irrelevant. "My intention," writes Proctor, "is not to argue that today's antitobacco efforts have fascist roots, or that public health measures are in principle totalitarian—as some libertarians seem to want us to believe."[90] Proctor's systematic labeling of Nazi health measures as "fascist" is as misleading as it is politically correct. Hitler was not a fascist and National Socialism was not a fascist movement. It was a socialist movement wrapped in the flag of nationalism. The terms "fascist" and "fascism" belong to Mussolini and his movement, and to Franco's, neither of which exhibited the kind of interest in health or genocide that was exhibited by Hitler and the Nazis.

Proctor steers clear of discussing psychiatric practices in Nazi Germany, such as the following typical episode, although they resemble closely psychiatric practices in the United States today. A father, a retired philologist, complains about the sudden death of his physically healthy schizophrenic son, Hans. He writes to the head of the institution where Hans had been confined, complaining that the explanation for his death was "contrary to the truth" and that "this affair appears to be rather murky." The psychiatrist replies: "The content of your letter . . . force[s] me to consider psychiatric measures against you. . . . should you continue to harass us with further communications, I shall be forced to have you examined by a public health physician."[91] Although Proctor's apologetics for pharmacracy in America diminishes the intellectual significance of his work, it does not impair the value of his documentation.

As Proctor himself shows, it was principally psychiatry that provided the "scientific" justification and personnel for medical mass murder in Nazi Germany. Nevertheless, he declares: "I should reassure the reader that I have no desire to efface the brute and simple facts—the complicity in crime or the sinister stupidities of Nazi ideology."[92] To call Nazi ideology "stupid" is like calling a distasteful religious belief "stupid." It is a self-righteous refusal to understand the other's ideology on its own terms, as if understanding it were tantamount to approving it. The truth is that the Nazi health ideology closely resembles the American health ideology. Each rests on the same premises—that the individual is incompetent to protect himself from himself and needs the protection of the paternalistic state, thus turning private health into public health. Proctor is too eager to efface the method in the madness of the Nazis's *furor therapeuticus politicus*, perhaps because it is so alarmingly relevant to our version of it.

"Nazism itself," he writes, "I will be treating as . . . a vast hygienic experiment designed to bring about an exclusionist sanitary utopia. That sanitary utopia was a vision not unconnected with *fascism's* [sic] more familiar genocidal aspects. . . ."[93] It was not fascism, which was not genocidal, but medical puritanism that motivated the Nazis to wage therapeutic wars against cancer and Jews. This is a crucial point. Once we begin to worship health as an all-pervasive good—a moral value that trumps all others, especially liberty—it becomes sanctified as a kind of secular holiness.

With respect to the relationship between health and the state, Hitler's basic goal was the same as Plato's, Aristotle's, and the modern public health zealots'—namely, abolishing the boundary between private and public health. Here are some striking examples, all of which Proctor misleadingly interprets as manifestations of "fascism":

- Your body belongs to the nation! Your body belongs to the Führer! You have the duty to be healthy! Food is not a private matter! (National Socialist slogans.)[94]

- We have the duty, if necessary, to die for the Fatherland; why should we not also have the duty to be healthy? Has the Führer not explicitly demanded this? (Antitobacco activist, 1939)[95]

- Nicotine damages not just the individual but the population as a whole. (Antitobacco activist, 1940)[96]

Hitler and his entourage were health fanatics obsessed with cleanliness and with killing "bugs," the latter category including unwanted people, especially Jews, Gypsies, homosexuals, and mental patients. Hitler neither drank nor smoked and was a vegetarian. Preoccupied with the fear of illness and the welfare of animals, he could not "tolerate the idea of animals' being killed for human consumption."[97] After Hitler became Chancellor, Reichsmarshall Hermann Göring announced an end to the "unbearable torture and suffering in animal experiments." The medical mass murder of mental patients went hand in hand with the prohibition of vivisection, which was declared a capital offense.[98] The fact that the Nazi public health ethic demanded not only respect for the health of the greatest numbers (of Aryans) but also for the health of animals (except "bugs") illustrates—as does also the work of bioethicist Peter Singer[99]—the connections between the love of pharmacracy and animal rights on one hand, and the loathing of human rights and the lives of imperfect persons on the other hand.

Instead of viewing the Nazi experience with medicalized politics as a cautionary tale illuminating the dangers lurking in the alliance between medicine and the state, Proctor uses it to speculate about what the Nazi war on cancer "tells us about the nature of *fascism.*"[100] He arrives at the comforting conclusion that "the Nazi analogy is pretty marginal to contemporary discussions about euthanasia" and criticizes "pro-tobacco activists"—as if opposing anti-tobacco legislation made one automatically a "pro-tobacco activist"—who "play the Nazi card."[101] Our future liberty, and health as well, may depend on whether we dismiss the analogy between pharmacracy in Nazi Germany and contemporary America as "pretty marginal," as Proctor believes we should, or whether, as I suggest, we view it as terrifyingly relevant and treat it with utmost seriousness.

MEDICALIZING "PSYCHOLOGICAL TRAUMA"

To future students of American history, 1999 may well seem like a peaceful year. This is not the way the medicalizers of life see it. "The world as we approach the millennium," intones a physician in *JAMA,* "is full of horrific events, in addition to warfare, that can lead to posttraumatic stress disorder (PTSD). Survivors of natural disasters and life-threatening violence, including recent attacks at schools, religious centers, and other venues not normally associated with bloodshed in the United States, may develop PTSD, *particularly if they do not receive immediate mental health care.*"[102]

Since the diagnosis of PTSD rests on the concept of trauma, we must be clear about what we mean when we use that term. *Webster's* primary definition of trauma is "an injury or wound to a living *body* caused by the application of *external force or violence*" (emphasis added). The diagnosis of PTSD, like that of mental illness itself, thus rests on metaphorizing the word "trauma," changing its meaning from physical injury to the body to psychological injury to the mind. Making the diagnosis does not require that the subject suffer an actual injury. Having *witnessed* a "traumatic situation" is enough. Every such witness is presumed to suffer from or is a candidate for PTSD, unless he receives prompt mental health care *to prevent it.*

PTSD is now routinely *imputed* to people, especially to children helpless to reject the label. A child is murdered or kills himself. Instantly, his classmates—perhaps all of the children in the school—become patient fodder for "grief counselors," forcibly imposed on them by the health care commissars of the therapeutic state.[103] Adults, too, are treated as if they could not manage their own grief unassisted by helpers they do not seek. A plane crashes. Relatives and friends of the victims are met by "grief counselors." What in the past Americans would have considered ugly meddling, they now accept as medically sound mental health care.

Madison was right when he warned his fellow Americans that of all the enemies to public liberty, war is "the most to be dreaded, because it . . . is the parent of armies." However, perhaps because he was so secure in being an adult, he ignored the infantilism that often clings to people throughout life, manifested by their love of soldiering and their adoration of military heroes. Socialist leaders love soldiers and the socialist masses love soldiering for them: "The Nazi state declared civil servants to be 'administrative soldiers,' school teachers 'soldiers of education,' doctors 'soldiers of medicine.' "[104] Soviet propaganda employed similar images. The American therapeutic state also loves soldiers—waging wars against diseases, drugs, and other "social problems," such as teenage pregnancy, suicide, violence, and war itself. Literal soldiers, sent abroad by the government, are "peace keepers" where there is no peace, and "liberators" where the term "liberty" means the opportunity to persecute and kill your adversary. Metaphorical soldiers—often led by arrogant and ignorant First Ladies—are people whose mantra Wystan Auden aptly satirized thus: "We are all here on earth to help others; what on earth the others are here for, I don't know."[105]

In the United States today, the indoctrination to help—actually, to judge, condemn, report, and stigmatize—other people's behavior, from relatives to schoolmates, begins in early childhood and never ceases. The view that certain disapproved or disliked behaviors are not necessarily "problems" and might not be the business of others is considered heresy. The individual as informant—"helping" others with their "health problems"—has become our ideal of the "responsible" person and model citizen. The fact that many such persons are unwilling or unable to assume responsibility for their own behavior only enhances their image.

It takes a lot of helpless people to keep all the helpers happy, and the helpers, thanks to their diligence and army of informants, are never at a loss to find people who are in dire need of their help. This is where medicalizing everyday life becomes useful. Most people have come to accept—apparently without anyone in a position to object—that bad deeds are due to diseases and hence the doer is blameless, while good deeds are due to free will and hence the doer deserves credit for them.

Posttraumatic Stress Disorder (PTSD)

The *DSM-IV* defines PTSD as a set of distressing feelings that follow "witnessing an event that involves death, injury, or other threat to the physical integrity of another person, or learning about unexpected or violent death, serious harm, or threat of death or injury by a family member or other close associate."[106] By this definition, the entire population of Europe between 1939 and 1945 was the victim of undiagnosed and untreated PTSD.

James M. Turnbull, a professor of family medicine at East Tennessee State University, warns physicians to be on the alert for PTSD among "battered women and men, adult children of alcoholics, police officers and firefighters, medical personnel who deal directly with trauma victims, noncombatants in war-torn areas such as—to choose just two recent ones—Kosovo and East Timor, and occasionally even spouses and children of persons with PTSD."[107] The mere act of living with someone with PTSD is here construed as a risk for contracting it. For good measure, Turnbull reembraces the traditional religious view of suicide as murder: "Grief following the suicide of a friend or relative presents a special case of emotional trauma. . . . A survivor's reaction during this time almost always includes . . . anger at the dead person, who is not only the victim but also the *killer* of the survivor's loved one."[108]

To the psychiatrically enlightened, anything connected with death is now a symptom of mental illness: thinking about death is "suicidal ideation," wanting to die is "being a suicidal risk," witnessing death is "PTSD." Since death is an integral part of life, the medicalization of death goes a long way toward creating an endless supply of patients in need of help. In the past, attending a funeral was a somber social custom, honoring the deceased and his relatives. Today, especially if the deceased is displayed in an open casket, it is "witnessing an event that involves death," hence a pathogen causing PTSD. A movie reviewer remarks: "In past ages, Joan [of Arc] has been seen as a mystic, a saint, a national hero. Now, in keeping with the times, she is a victim of post-traumatic stress disorder."[109]

Because mental patients often kill themselves, psychiatric residents are especially prone to become victims of PTSD: 20 percent report symptoms of it after patient suicide. "My first reaction," says [Cindy] Grief [*sic*], after one of her patients killed herself, "was to tell myself that she had a disease like cancer and that it was her illness that caused her death." Although that is part of the psychiatric catechism she was taught, it did not help: soon she was named in a lawsuit brought by the family.[110] Psychiatric residents are upset after a patient's suicide because they are not taught that killing oneself is a basic human right and incarcerating people in mental hospitals is a grave moral wrong; and that, although the suicide is not their fault (because it is not in their power to prevent it), when a mental patient kills himself, his "loved ones" and the lawyers they hire are likely to interpret the act as *prima facie* evidence of the psychiatrist's having committed medical malpractice.[111]

HEALTH ÜBER ALLES

Clearly, many Americans believe that the coercive medical control of most (bad) behaviors is justified and proper, because they are diseases, or are caused by diseases, or are the causes of diseases. Barry R. Bloom, dean of the Harvard School of Public Health, states: "The real culprits behind heart disease, cancer, stroke, and injuries are *the underlying causes* of these conditions—tobacco use (leading to 19 percent of all deaths), unhealthy diet and inactivity (14 percent), alcohol (5 percent), infectious disease (5 percent), firearms (about 2 percent), and accidents (1 percent)."[112] What, one wonders, will people die of after all the preventable causes of diseases have been prevented?

When Health Trumps Liberty

When health is equated with freedom, liberty as a political concept vanishes. We understand and accept the person who prefers security over liberty, but we do not understand or accept the person who prefers disease over health, death over life.

In 1999, at the 11th World Congress of the World Psychiatric Association, Benedetto Saraceno, M.D., director of the WHO's department of mental health, urged psychiatrists "to embrace a conceptual shift that expands on the traditional boundaries of psychiatry . . . [and] serve people affected by violent conflicts, civil wars, and disasters . . . and displaced people, many of whom will suffer from anxiety disorders, depression, and substance abuse."[113] (I am not aware of a psychiatric leader ever urging his colleagues to contract the traditional boundaries of psychiatry.) The pharmacrats' agenda, based on the new *coercive-therapeutic concept of disease*, differs radically from the medical scientist's agenda, based on the old *noncoercive-pathological concept of disease.* To advance their agenda, the pharmacrats shift the focus, their own and the public's, from phenomenon to tactic, from objectively demonstrable *disease* to dramatically advertised *prevention and treatment.*

The medical doctor treats cancer of the lung. The political doctor treats smoking, preventable by legislation, litigation, and taxation, and curable with nicotine, administered by any route other than inhalation. Sanctimony and hypocrisy replace honesty and self-discipline. The Renaissance popes preached celibacy and fornicated. Political doctors preach zero tolerance for tobacco and smoke. At the 52nd World Health Assembly, Surgeon General David Satcher publicly whined: "I was personally concerned to see delegates from many countries smoking . . . allowing harmful exposure of UN employees, visitors, and delegates to environmental tobacco smoke, a known carcinogen."[114] Satcher did not engage in a more meaningful protest at the convention, such as walking out of smoke-filled rooms, nor did he propose a more meaningful protest in the pages of *JAMA*.

Suicide prevention is another, perhaps the most dramatic, example of coercion masquerading as care. In September 1999, Surgeon General Satcher declared "suicide a serious public health threat" and proposed "educating the public to recognize when someone seems 'at risk' for suicide and how to better help that person get help. That includes doctors and nurses, but also the clergy and others who interact with people and hear about their problems. *We want coaches, we want schoolteachers, we want hairdressers* [to be informants]." [115] Satcher's spokesman explained: "It's simple, it's understandable, and there's *near universal agreement* that these 15 steps can prevent suicide."[116] Recognizing that the term "suicide prevention" is a euphemism for psychiatric coercion is taboo; rejecting the premise that all suicide ought to be prevented is unthinkable. Satcher's antisuicide proposals—like the wars on drugs and smoking—reek of hypocrisy. He must know that the suicide rate among physicians is two to three times that among the general public.

THE STATIST-SOCIALIST BIAS IN HEALTH-CARE THINKING

Throughout this book I have touched on the statist-socialist bias that underlies much of the discussion about health-care policy and public health, exemplified by Nobel Laureate Kenneth J. Arrow's dictum: "It is the general social consensus, clearly, that the *laissez-faire* solution for medicine is intolerable."[117]

The way we think about medical care and the language we use to talk about it are themselves problematic and deserving of attention. Health care planners think in terms of *other people's needs*, determined by physicians or politicians. Patients think in terms of their *own wants*, determined by them. People buy health care *not because they want health care, but because they do not want to be sick.* This negative motivation creates a more intense consumer dependence on authority for health care than for other goods and services. On whose authority can or should the consumer depend? The physician's? The medical profession's? The government's? For the better part of the twentieth century, it was not enough that the practicing physician be well trained. He also had to be *licensed by the state.* Medical licensure *by the states* was supposed to guarantee the public a high level of physician competence and thus of medical care. By the end of the twentieth century, most Americans concluded, probably without giving the matter much thought, that this was not enough, that the time had come to place their trust for the provision of reliable medical care in the *federal government.*

We have come to take our dependence on the federal government for *health protection* so much for granted that we no longer notice how it has infected the way we speak and think about *prohibitions* imposed on us by the state. On December 28, 1999, President Clinton proposed "a new initiative to *protect consumers from the illegal sale* of pharmaceuticals over the Internet." The proposed regulation, designed to protect "unsuspecting consumers [who] may fall prey to fly-by-night Internet pharmacies . . . [will] identify, investigate, and *prosecute websites selling such items as: prescription drugs without a valid prescription.*"[118] This is typical pharmacratic newspeak. The consumers Clinton offers to "protect" cannot be *unsuspecting* if they know how to use a computer and the Internet, nor can they be *prey* to unscrupulous vendors if their aim is to free themselves of the constraints of our prescription-drug laws. Depriving people of the opportunity to evade our draconian drug laws is here portrayed as an act of liberation-protection from health fraud. Pharmacratic controls may yet prove to be the Achilles heel of the unregulated Internet.

Loving Leviathan: Deifying and Medicalizing the State

The belief that providing health care to people is a function of the state is a part of the view of the state as a secular God. A few examples of the deification of the state, foreign and American, should suffice here.[119]

In 1928, Grigori Pyatakov, a Soviet leader, declared: "According to Lenin, the Communist Party is based on the principle of coercion which doesn't recognize any limitations or inhibitions . . . moral, political, or even physical. Such a Party is capable of achieving miracles."[120] In 1997, a French Communist official justified the Soviet Union's murdering millions of its own citizens as follows: "Agreed, both Nazis and communists killed. But while Nazis killed from hatred of humanity, the communists killed from love."[121]

The deification of the state was and is as popular in the United States as it was and is in Europe. In 1916, John Dewey, declared: "The question of the limits of individual powers, or liberties, or rights, is finally a question of the most efficient use of means for ends. . . . [Some] forms of *liberty may be obstructive.*"[122] Alexander Meiklejohn—a less-well-known but perhaps more influential political philosopher—abjured personal liberty more subtly but perhaps even more deeply. In 1935, he wrote that "Life, Liberty, and Property . . . may even be taken away [by the government] provided that the action by which this is done is justly and properly performed."[123] And in 1960, he declared: "Political freedom does not mean freedom from control. It means self-control."[124] Tito put it more simply: "The more powerful the State, the more freedom."[125] The pharmacratic version of this maxim becomes: "The more powerful Medicine, the more health, and the more health, the more freedom."

The socialization of health care in the United States is, for all practical purposes, a *fait accompli*. However, that reality has been obscured by the absence of a directly nationalized ("socialized") system of health care, as well as by the American system's being decked out with the vocabulary of choice, market competition, and patient autonomy. The result is deeply ironic: the more thoroughly socialized our health-care system becomes, the more physicians and patients alike complain that its shortcomings lie in its capitalistic excesses.

Health policy expert Dan E. Beauchamp writes: "When I came to New York in 1988, my view of health care reform was captured in the image of the 'big wave' that would *transform everything, not only altering health care from a private to a social good but permanently reshaping the body politic, enlarging the communal sphere.*"[126] Like a good Jacobin, Beauchamp dreamed of a "universal health care . . . to change people and politics."[127] Beauchamp acknowledges that he is not interested in improving anyone's *private health*. "I began this task [formulating health care policy]," he writes, "seeking to translate the public health viewpoint into the language of social justice and equality, suggesting that 'public health,' not 'health care' should be the primary or basic good."[128] Beauchamp is not interested in improving the health of any particular person as that person might want to improve it. To the contrary, he is interested in depriving individuals of their freedom to use their own funds to purchase medical care. "Republican equality would limit the power of money . . . over health policy . . . [and would limit] liberty to protect the health and safety of citizens as a body, the *public health—a central goal of all republican schemes of government.*"[129]

Having said this, Beauchamp denies that he wants to abridge liberty by redefining freedom as the protection of the collective from disease: "The idea of liberty should mean, above all else, the liberation of society from the injustices of preventable disability and early death. . . . extending life and health to all persons will require some diminution of personal choices . . . such restrictions are not only fair and do not constitute abridgment of fundamental liberties, they are a basic sign and imprint of a just society and a guarantee of the most basic of all freedoms—protection against man's most ancient foe." [130] According to Beauchamp, the market is a "prison [that] diminishes justice. . . . The truth of the market rests on a private and *interested* view. The truth of the political sphere rests on a more general and *disinterested* view."[131] He concludes: "Giving everyone roughly the same level of care based on their need makes everyone aware that they are equals."[132] This is a proposal to use health-care policy to justify political coercion in the service of a dystopian goal that has no relation whatever to health as a medical concept. Finally, taking the New Deal as his model for social engineering, Beauchamp prescribes for us our state-religion: "Our myth for the next American republic should be that *we do things together in order to live together.* This new myth would build on the New Deal and its ideal of national community."[133] What we need, in short, is a New Leviathan led by a medical Führer—"a new leader who battles on behalf of the people and launches the last big wave of reform, putting in place a powerful new institution that secures our health care future and much else besides."[134]

In a similar vein, Howard Waitzkin, professor of medicine at the University of New Mexico, advocates re-forming America's medical services along explicitly socialist lines. In his book, *The Second Sickness,* he explains: "Under capitalism, illness is exploited for a variety of purposes by a number of groups, including profit-making corporations, health care professionals, and medical centers."[135] Waitzkin's excuse for alcoholism illustrates the meshing of the psychiatric and socialist perspectives on drug abuse. "Alcoholism [according to Engels] was rooted finally in social structure; the attribution of responsibility to the individual worker was misguided."[136] Americans have accepted this viewpoint without any recognition of its pseudoscientific, Marxist roots.

Like Beauchamp, Waitzkin is more interested in creating "state power" and eliminating private medicine than in letting individuals choose the kind of health care they prefer. Physicians, Waitzkin declares, "hold class interests that often impede progress toward a more egalitarian distribution of goods and services. Doctors, like bankers and corporate managers, possess economic advantages and customary life styles that they do not willingly sacrifice on behalf of the poor."[137] Waitzkin evidently believes that degrading the rich would elevate the poor. The Soviet experience, one would have thought, has decisively disproved this fantasy, but not in Waitzkin's socialist construction of reality: "The Soviet Union eliminated its chronic problems of epidemics and cut its infant mortality rate by more than half in one generation."[138] The Soviet Union also succeeded in increasing its adult mortality rate, reducing the life expectancy of its citizens by some two decades below that of people in the West or in Japan.

Most academic physicians now champion statist medicine as the embodiment of a higher, altruistic morality. Leon Eisenberg, a professor of psychiatry at Harvard, calls Milton Friedman "the high priest of laissez-faire capitalism," as if capitalism were self-evidently sinful, and concludes his plea for socialist medicine with this self-flattering outcry: "Will we try to save our skins by delivering minimally adequate care on the cheap or will we stand up and be counted in the fight for universal health insurance?"[139]

The right-thinking physician is now an advocate of merging medicine and the state. He does not call this "socialized medicine," a tabooed phrase. He calls it the "single-payer" systems or "universal health care coverage." Speaking at a meeting in January 2000, Arnold Relman, the former editor in chief of the *New England Journal of Medicine*, endorsed "three examples of single payers: Britain, Canada, and U.S. Medicare. One advantage, he stated, was physician autonomy: British and Canadian doctors are 'free to do what they want with the resources provided.' U.S. Medicare, which [according to Relman] 'is not socialized at all, exerts virtually no control over the practice of medicine.' "[140] Marcia Angell, editor in chief of the *New England Journal of Medicine*, declares: "In a 1993 editorial, . . . I called for a universal, single-payer system and suggested that we could attain that goal by extending Medicare to all Americans. . . . Medicare is far more efficient than the market-based part of our health care system."[141] Herbert Pardes, president of New York–Presbyterian Healthcare System, complains: "Academic medicine has been turned over to the marketplace and treated like a product. We need universal health care coverage to help both *indigent people and the institutions that serve them*."[142]

Relman's views sound like nothing so much as the enthusiastic reports of liberals returning from their visits to the Soviet Union in the 1930s. The "single-payer" system—which Angell calls "market-based"—has, of course, not the remotest similarity to what classical liberals call a "free market." Finally, Pardes recommends that we return to the health-care system of the 1940s, with this difference: *every patient* should be in the same position of economic-existential dependence on the system in which the charity patient used to be.

CONCLUSIONS

The collectivization of American medicine, like the collectivization of much else in America, began during the presidency of Franklin D. Roosevelt. In 1940, in a speech delivered at the dedication of the newly established National Institutes of Health, Roosevelt declared: "The defense this nation seeks involves a great deal more than building airplanes, ships, guns, and bombs. We cannot be a strong nation unless we are a healthy nation."[143] With equal justification, Roosevelt might have said: "We cannot be a strong nation unless we are a prosperous nation."

We have become a prosperous nation by separating the economy and the state, not by making the state the source of employment, as have the communists, with the disastrous results we are familiar with. We can become a healthy nation only by separating medicine and the state, not by making the state the source of health care, as have the Communists, with the disastrous results we are familiar with.

Long before the reign of modern totalitarianisms, English economist and statesman Richard Cobden (1804–1865) warned: "They who propose to influence by force the traffic of the world, forget that affairs of trade, like matters of conscience, change their very nature if touched by the hand of violence; for as faith, if forced, would no longer be religion, but hypocrisy, so commerce becomes robbery if coerced by warlike armaments."[144] The same principle applies to medicine: As "affairs of trade . . . change their very nature if touched by the hand of violence," so affairs of medicine also change their very nature if touched by the hand of violence and, if forced, cease to be forms of treatment and, instead, become forms of tyranny.

Americans' love affair with pharmacracy now transcends traditional distinctions between left and right, liberal and conservative, Democrat and Republican.[145] Even Libertarians are often indifferent to the dangers posed by Leviathan, provided it has an M.D. degree and prescribes drugs.[146] Physicians, who ought to know better but for the most part don't, are perhaps the most naive and at the same time the most zealous advocates of medical interventions for all manner of human problems. Writing in *JAMA*, two physicians plead for a "comprehensive public health surveillance of firearm injuries." Why? Because "firearm injuries are a leading cause of death and disability in the United States."[147] We are building a society based on the false premise that if X is a "leading cause" of death, then X is a disease and a public health problem whose prevention and treatment justify massive infringements on personal freedom.

Clearly, the leading cause of death is being alive. The therapeutic state thus swallows up everything human, on the seemingly rational ground that nothing falls outside the province of health and medicine, just as the theological state had swallowed up everything human, on the perfectly rational ground that nothing falls outside the province of God and religion. Lest it seem that I exaggerate the parallels between these two total states and the religious nature of the therapeutic state, consider Vice President Al Gore's by-no-means-atypical remarks, offered in an address at Emory University on June 1, 2000. Pledging to wage the war on cancer with renewed vigor, he declared: "Within ten years, no one in America should have to die from colon cancer, breast cancer, or prostate cancer. . . . The power to fight cancer comes from the heart and from the human spirit. But most of all, it comes from being able to imagine a day when you are cancer-free." His website carried his message under the banner headline "Gore Sets Goal for a Cancer Free-America."[148] Thus do Christian Science and the wars on diseases blend into political vapidity and pharmacratic tyranny.

Since much of the work of the pharmacrats entails legislation, regulation, and coercion, the need for lawyers expands even more rapidly than does the need for doctors. The steady increase in the number of lawyers compared to the number of physicians is consistent both with the expansion of pharmacratic tyranny and with the underlying conflict between health and freedom that so many people sense. In 1956, approximately 7,500 law degrees and 6,000 medical degrees were awarded in the United States for a ratio of 1.2 law degrees for every M.D. In 1996, 40,000 law degrees and 15,000 medical degrees were awarded, for a ratio of 2.6.[149]

America's drift toward pharmacracy has not escaped the attention of perceptive social commentators. "Our politicians," observes Andrew Ferguson, "are transcending politics. . . . How is it . . . that politicians who for years promised to keep government out of our bedrooms now see fit to invite their way into our souls? They have cast themselves as empaths; soul-fixing is their job. . . . Their bet is that America today wants a Therapist in Chief."[150] Indeed, the medical metaphors regularly used by our leaders—and their wives and cabinet members—have made them seem such.

Actually, I believe Americans want a therapist in chief who is both physician and priest—an authority that will protect them from having to assume responsibility not only for their own health care but also for their behaviors that make them ill, literally or figuratively. Pandering to this passion, politicians assure them they have a "right to health" and that their maladies are "no-fault diseases"; promise them a "patient's bill of rights" and an America "free of cancer" and "free of drugs"; and stupefy them with an inexhaustible torrent of mind-altering prescription drugs and mind-numbing antidisease and antidrug propaganda—as if anyone could be *for* illness or drug abuse.

Formerly, people rushed to embrace totalitarian states. Now they rush to embrace the therapeutic state. When they discover that the therapeutic state is about tyranny, not therapy, it will be too late.

EPILOGUE

Well then, maybe it would be worth mentioning the three periods of history. When man believed that happiness was dependent upon God, he killed for religious reasons. When he believed that happiness was dependent upon the form of government, he killed for political reasons. . . . After dreams that were too long, true nightmares . . . we arrived at the present period of history. Man woke up, discovered that which we always knew, that happiness is dependent upon health, and began to kill for therapeutic reasons. . . . It is medicine that has come to replace both religion and politics in our time.

Adolfo B. Casares[1]

Although we have little to fear from the traditional foes of freedom, commentators across the political spectrum lament the creeping loss of our liberties. How can this be?

- Our foreign policies have not failed: America is more secure than ever from foreign aggression.

- Our religious policies have not failed: The clergy has no power to deprive anyone of liberty.

- Our economic policies have not failed: More Americans are working and are economically more secure than ever before.

Epilogue

How, then, have we failed to protect our liberties? By entrusting the care of our health to the state and thus falling into the very error against which Frederick Bastiat (1801–1850), the French economist and political philosopher, warned more than 150 years ago. He wrote:

> When we oppose subsidies, we are charged with opposing the very thing that it was proposed to subsidize and of being the enemies of all kinds of activity, because we want these activities to be voluntary and to seek their proper reward in themselves. Thus, if we ask that the state not intervene, by taxation, in religious matters, we are atheists. If we ask that the state not interfere, by taxation, in education, then we hate enlightenment. . . . If we think that the state should not subsidize artists, we are barbarians who judge the arts useless. I protest with all my power against these inferences. Far from entertaining the absurd thought of abolishing religion, education, property, labor, and the arts, when we ask the state to protect the free development of all these types of human activity without keeping them on the payroll *at one another's expense*, we believe, on the contrary, that all these vital forces of society should develop harmoniously under the influence of liberty and that none of them should become, as we see has happened today, a source of trouble, abuses, tyranny, and disaster. Our adversaries believe that an activity that is neither subsidized nor regulated is abolished. We believe the contrary. Their faith is in the legislator, not in mankind. Ours is in mankind, not in the legislator.[2]

These words are astonishingly timely. After vanquishing the two great twentieth-century statisms—National Socialism and Communism—we are sacrificing our freedom on the altar of the most catholic and democratic of all modern statisms, the ideology of pharmacracy embodied in the therapeutic state guaranteeing every man, woman, and child a "right to health care."

Patrick Henry's famous cry "Give me liberty, or give me death!" dramatizes the potential conflict between liberty and life. Many people may not be willing to go as far as Henry, but at least they recognize the dilemma. With no similar tradition alerting us to the potential conflict between liberty and the worship of health, we are blind to the dangers such worship poses. What happens when we must choose between liberty and health? In a 1998 Gallup poll, 62 percent of the respondents agreed that in order to reduce drug use, they "would be willing to give up some freedoms."[3] Let us not be deceived by slogans: The term "drug use" is a misnomer for what Mark Twain called "other people's bad habits." Abstaining from smoking or drinking neither requires nor entails giving up one's freedoms. Forcing others to do so is another matter.

Epilogue

The evidence presented in this book confirms that most Americans indeed prefer health—or at least what they think is "health"—over liberty, forgetting Benjamin Franklin's warning, "They that can give up essential liberty to obtain a little temporary safety, deserve neither liberty nor safety." Franklin recognized that those who give up liberty for safety obtain neither. We fail to recognize that by giving up liberty to obtain medical care, we lose both.

The first casualty of all wars is clear thinking and personal independence, replaced by the collective stupidity and timidity of a people united by fear and hatred against a common enemy. This sacrifice of liberty is perceived as liberation, whether the enemy is Communism or cancer. Day after day, in myriad ways we are no longer even conscious of, we choose health over freedom—and view our lack of free access to doctors and drugs as not a loss of liberty but a gain of affordable health care and protection from disease-producing dangers. The controversial slogan "better red than dead" has metamorphosed into the uncontroversial maxim "better to lose our freedom than endanger our health." The change in the *Zeitgeist* is more momentous than we realize.

A hundred years ago, in the glory days of bacteriology, physicians experimented on themselves in the interests of science. Today, in the glory days of medical ethics, they experiment on patients in the interests of the state. The physician experimenting on himself, especially with drugs, is considered a mentally deranged drug abuser and dealt with accordingly. The physician experimenting on others, especially mental patients without their consent, is considered a sophisticated neuroscientist and honored as a humanitarian.[4]

Both freedom and health are important values. That, precisely, is what makes their potential incompatibility an important moral issue. Sadly, the conflict is now entirely one-sided: everyone is on the side of health, as if it were synonymous with liberty. This is probably why no politician warns us, as did Patrick Henry, that we must choose between our political heritage of individual liberty and the utopian pharmacratic policies pursued by politicians of all stripes.

America's traditional political symbol is the Statue of Liberty, gracing the entrance to America's premier harbor, promising freedom to the oppressed. She has been eclipsed by a new symbol, the Surgeon General in full regalia—flanked by President, First Lady, and Drug Czar—promising to relieve people of the burden of caring for their bodies, minds, and hence their very lives as free and responsible adults.

Every American recognizes that when the government controls religion, all religion becomes state religion. But few Americans are willing to accept that when the government controls health, all health becomes public health and all privacy is lost. The erosion of our liberties is not a mystery. It is largely the result of the frightening alliance between medicine and the state, intensifying people's dependency on pharmacratic authority—fostered by, and in turn fostering, an expansive definition of disease covering all the vicissitudes of life.

A hundred years ago, physicians were therapeutic nihilists. They were right: there was little chance that a patient would benefit from a professional encounter with a physician. Today, physicians are therapeutic utopians. They are wrong: although patients often benefit from their professional encounters with a physician, sooner or later everyone dies.[5] The effort to eradicate disease is a quixotic quest. Not everyone thinks so. "Why," asks Emil Freireich, at the University of Texas Medical Center, "should anyone in good conscience . . . imagine that death is a part of life? . . . If we can understand disease and manipulate it, then I think one of the options that people must consider for themselves is the possibility of life forever."[6]

Absurd? In January 2000, the front cover of the *New York Times Magazine* boldly titled its feature essay: "Racing toward Immortality (or at Least Your 150th Birthday)."[7] Respected *New York Times* columnist William Safire opines: "In the millennium to come a curious question will occupy the minds of our descendants. It seems almost nutty to ask it today, but tomorrow's question will be: Why die? . . . For future people, doddering will no longer be an option. . . . for those readers of a distant tomorrow who will flip back through the millennia to access the *New York Times Archive*, one will say, 'You know, this fellow was incredibly prescient.' "[8] I doubt it.

The idea that physicians will liquidate disease and death is characteristic of the contemporary fashion in pharmacratic thinking. Medical professionals, politicians, and the public are in the grips of a delusionary, imperialist-utopian quest—a veritable modern crowd madness—that is at once the cause and the consequence of a naively medicalized view of life and death. One of the symptoms of this crowd madness is the widespread belief that every medical problem can be solved if we spend enough money on "research." In January 2000, at the Super Bowl in Atlanta, an advertisement displayed "A computer-faked image of Christopher Reeve [who is paraplegic] rising to his feet and walking. . . . Reeve . . . insisted that the scene in the commercial is 'something that can actually happen. Most scientists agree that with enough money and talent focused on spinal cord repair, the goal of [paraplegics] walking within the foreseeable future is a very real possibility.' "[9] We have replaced the false promise of a religious paradise in an afterlife with the false promise of a medical paradise in this life.

There are more dangerous possibilities lurking in this kind of utopian fantasy, such as the mania for curing "patients" regardless of their wishes and the killing of persons under the guise of suicide as "treatment." Most importantly, therapeutic zealotry fosters the erroneous belief that a *medical diagnosis is a moral justification for a medical treatment.* It is not. In a free society, *medical treatment is contingent on, and justified by, the patient's consent, not the physician's diagnostic "verdict."*

People in modern societies increasingly perceive health care as the supreme *political good.* The inevitable result is the gradual erosion of contract and the rule of law and their replacement by therapy and the rule of benefit.[10] In the therapeutic state, treatment is contingent on, and justified by, the diagnosis of the patient's illness and the physician's prescription of the proper remedy for it. With astonishing prescience, Goethe anticipated such a "humanistic medicalization" of life. He wrote: "I believe that in the end humanitarianism will triumph, but I fear that, at the same time, the world will become a big hospital, each person acting as the other's humane nurse."[11]

After World War I, Jules Romains, the once-famous French novelist and playwright, satirized the collectivist-coercive ideology of modern medicine by putting these words into the mouth of his protagonist, Dr. Knock: "It's a matter of principle with me to regard the entire population as our patients. . . . 'Health' is a word we could just as well erase from our vocabularies. . . . If you think it over, you'll be struck by its relation to the admirable concept of the nation in arms, a concept from which our modern states derive their strength."[12]

For centuries, the theocratic state exercised authority and used force in the name of God. Today, the therapeutic state exercises authority and uses force in the name of health. The reformers protested against prostituting the dominant, Roman Catholic, theology to satisfy the church's voracious appetite for power, because they disapproved of the theology. When the theology was of the reformers' own making, as in Calvin's Geneva, their opposition to theocracy vanished.

The Founders sought to protect the American people from the religious tyranny of the state, regardless of the religion. They did not anticipate, and could not have anticipated, that one day medicine would become a religion and that an alliance between medicine and the state would then threaten personal liberty and responsibility exactly as they had been threatened by an alliance between church and state.

I protest against prostituting medicine *or* religion—the treatment of bodies *and* the cure of souls—to satisfy the modern state's voracious appetite for power. The Founders faced the challenge of separating the cure of souls by priests from the control of people by politicians. We face the challenge of separating the treatment of patients by medical doctors from the control of citizens by agents of the state pretending to be therapists.

NOTES

Complete references for books are listed in the Bibliography.

PREFACE

1. Aristotle, *Politica (Politics)*, (1337.a), p. 1305.
2. Quoted in J. Sanders, "The tyranny of the proper," *The Freeman,* 48: 757–758 (December) 1998, p. 757.
3. G. K. Chesterton, "Broadcast talk" (6–11–35), http://www.the700club. org/bibleresources/theology/chesterton.
4. Quoted in J. Sullum, "To your health!" *National Review*, September 13, 1999, pp. 66– 67; p. 67, emphasis added.
5. "Cindy McCain's own story," *Newsweek,* November 15, 1999, p. 49.
6. E. Thomas, "The woman by his side," *Newsweek*, February 14, 2000, p. 34.
7. T. S. Szasz, *Fatal Freedom*, pp. 80–86.
8. T. S. Szasz, *Ceremonial Chemistry*, p. 139.
9. Ibid.

ACKNOWLEDGMENTS

1. S. Butler, quoted in R. V. Sampson, *The Psychology of Power*, p. 110.

INTRODUCTION: WHAT COUNTS AS A DISEASE?

1. S. Johnson, "Preface to the Dictionary," in S. Johnson, *Johnson's Dictionary*, p. 26.

2. G. K. Chesterton, *The Quotable Chesterton*, p. 368.

3. T. S. Szasz, *Law, Liberty, and Psychiatry* and *The Manufacture of Madness.*

CHAPTER 1. MEDICINE: FROM GNOSTIC HEALING TO EMPIRICAL SCIENCE

1. J. C. Traupman, *The New College Latin and English Dictionary.*

2. Job 2:6–7.

3. Ibid., 5:17–18, emphasis added.

4. L. N. Magner, *A History of Medicine,* pp. 1, 3.

5. Ibid., p. 71.

6. See especially T. Szasz, *The Myth of Psychotherapy* and *Ceremonial Chemistry.*

7. B.C.H. Harvey, "Anatomy, Gross," in *Encyclopaedia Britannica*, vol. 1, pp. 870, 871.

8. R. Ghys, "Medicine in the past millennium" (Letter), *New England Journal of Medicine*, 342: 1367 (May 4), 2000.

9. C. C. Mettler and F. A. Mettler, *History of Medicine.*

10. Molière, *The Misanthrope and Other Plays*; J. Romains, *Knock*; T. Mann, *Confessions of Felix Krull.*

11. N. Guterman, *The Anchor Book of Latin Quotations*, pp. 52, 53.

12. T. S. Szasz, *Fatal Freedom.*

13. T. S. Szasz, *Insanity.*

CHAPTER 2. SCIENTIFIC MEDICINE: DISEASE

1. R. Virchow, "Concerning standpoints in scientific medicine," in A. L. Caplan, H. T. Engelhardt, Jr., and J. J. McCartney, eds., *Concepts of Health and Disease*, pp. 188–190, p. 188.

2. A. R. Feinstein, *Clinical Judgment*, pp. 109, 111.

3. J. Roosen et al., "Comparison of premortem clinical diagnoses in critically ill patients and subsequent autopsy findings," *Proceedings of the Mayo Clinic*, 75: 562–567 (June), 2000; p. 562.

4. J. Selden, quoted in K. Thomas, *Religion and the Decline of Magic*, p. 435.

5. Exodus 9:8–9.

6. "Anthrax," *Encyclopaedia Britannica*, vol. 2, pp. 34–35.

7. J. Kroll and B. Bachrach, "Sin and the etiology of disease in pre-Crusade Europe," *Journal of the History of Medicine and Allied Sciences*, 41: 395–414 (October), 1986; V. Nutton, "The seeds of disease: An explanation of contagion and infection from the Greeks to the Renaissance," *Medical History*, 27: 1–34, 1983.

8. H. Cohen, "The evolution of the concept of disease," in B. Lush, ed., *Concepts of Medicine*, pp. 159–169.

9. S. L. Robbins, *Pathologic Basis of Disease*, p. 1.

10. Quoted in G. Canguilhem, *On the Normal and the Pathological*, p. 46.

11. E. Rubin and J. L. Farber, *Pathology*, p. 2.

12. A. R. Feinstein, *Clinical Judgment*, p. 119.

13. D. M. Reese, "Fundamentals: Rudolf Virchow and modern medicine," *Western Journal of Medicine*, 169: 105–108, 1998.

14. E. H. Ackerknecht, *Rudolf Virchow*, p. v.

15. B. A. Boyd, *Rudolf Virchow*, p. 15, emphasis added.

16. R. Virchow, "Concerning standpoints in scientific medicine" (1847), in A. L. Caplan, H. T. Engelhardt, Jr., and J. J. McCartney, eds., *Concepts of Health and Disease*, pp. 188–190, p. 188, emphasis added.

17. R. Virchow, "One hundred years of general pathology," in A. L. Caplan, H. T. Engelhardt, Jr., and J. J. McCartney, eds., *Concepts of Health and Disease*, pp. 190–195, p. 190, emphasis added.

18. Ibid., pp. 192–193.

19. R. J. Dubos, *Louis Pasteur*, p. 243.

20. B. A. Boyd, *Rudolf Virchow*, p. 50.

21. H. G. Schlumberger, "Rudolf Virchow, revolutionist," *Annals of Medical History*, 4: 147–153, 1942.

22. B. A. Boyd, *Rudolf Virchow*, pp. 146, 158.

23. E. H. Ackerknecht, *Rudolf Virchow*, pp. 131–132.

24. B. A. Boyd, *Rudolf Virchow*, p. 140.

25. R. J. Dubos, *Louis Pasteur*, p. 122.

26. Ibid., p. 218.

27. Ibid., p. 221.

28. Ibid., p. 162.

29. Quoted in ibid., p. 267.

30. "Bassi, Agostino" in *Encyclopaedia Britannica*, vol. 3, pp. 260–261.

31. R. J. Dubos, *Louis Pasteur*, p. 210.

32. Ibid., pp. 213–214.

33. Ibid., emphasis added.

34. Ibid., p. 257.

35. Quoted in ibid., p. 267.

36. See Chapter 7 for further discussion.

37. L. R. Kass, *Toward a More Natural Science*, p. 173.

38. J. Roosen et al., "Comparison of premortem clinical diagnoses in critically ill patients and subsequent autopsy findings," *Proceedings of the Mayo Clinic*, 75: 562–567 (June), 2000, pp. 562, 567.

39. G. W. Moore and G. M. Hutchins, "The persistent importance of autopsies" (Editorial), *Proceedings of the Mayo Clinic*, 75: 557–558 (June), 2000, p. 557.

40. See, for example, D. France, "An inconvenient woman: In order to turn the murdered soldier Barry Winchell into a martyr for gay rights, activists first had to turn his girlfriend, Calpernia Addams, back into a man," *New York Times Magazine*, May 28, 2000, pp. 24–29.

41. T. Stuttaford, "Medical Briefing: Genetics is only proof of gender," *Times* (London), August 4, 1999, Internet edition. Copyright 1999 Times Newspapers Ltd.

42. R. S. Cotran, V. Kumar, T. Collins, and S. L. Robbins, eds. *Robbins Pathologic Basis of Disease*, 6th ed., p. 1.

43. See Chapter 5.

CHAPTER 3. CLINICAL MEDICINE: DIAGNOSIS

1. J. C. Bennett and F. Plum, "Medicine as a learned and humane profession," in J. C. Bennett and F. Plum, eds., *Cecil Textbook of Medicine*, 10th ed., vol. 1, p. 1.

2. R. P. Feynman, *"What Do You Care What Other People Think?"* p. 14. See also L. Lebovici, "Alternative (complementary) medicine: A cuckoo in the nest of empiricist reed warblers," *British Journal of Medicine*, 319: 1629–1631 (18–25 December), 1999.

3. F. Vinicor, "When is diabetes diabetes?" *JAMA*, 281: 1222–1224 (April 7), 1999; p. 1222.

4. A. R. Feinstein, *Clinical Judgment*, pp. 123 and 109, 111.

5. T. Szasz, "Diagnoses are not diseases," *The Lancet* (London), 338: 1574–1576 (December 21/28), 1991; and, generally, *Insanity*.

6. S. Freud, "An autobiographical study," [1924], in *SE*, vol. 20, pp. 1–76, p.12.

7. See Chapter 5.

8. M. Cottle, "Selling shyness: How doctors and drug companies created the 'social phobia' epidemic," *The New Republic*, August 2, 1999, p. 25.

9. R. A. Aronowitz, *Making Sense of Illness*, p. 7.

10. M. Clements and D. Hales, "In a new national survey, *Parade* asked: How healthy are we?" *Parade*, September 7, 1997, pp. 4–7, p. 4, emphasis added.

11. A. Marsh, "Business services: Express Scrips," *Forbes*, January 10, 2000, p. 92.

12. M. Cottle, "Selling shyness: How doctors and drug companies created the 'social phobia' epidemic," *The New Republic*, August 2, 1999, pp. 24–29, p. 26.

13. Examples abound. See, for example, D. Seligman, "The addiction made me do it," *Forbes*, May 29, 2000, pp. 102–103.

14. Associated Press, "Inmate sues for sex change," *New York Times*, January 8, 2000, Internet edition.

15. P. Hoch, quoted in L. R. Frank, ed., *Random House Webster's Quotationary*, p. 786.

16. See H. Ritvo, *The Platypus and the Mermaid*.

17. A. Moscovit, *Our Choice and History*, p. 177.

18. "Philip IV," in *Encyclopaedia Britannica*, vol. 17, pp. 835–836.

19. S. Wessely, "Responding to mass psychogenic illness" (Editorial), *New England Journal of Medicine*, 342: 129–130 (January 13), 2000.

20. T. F. Jones et al., "Mass psychogenic illness attributed to toxic exposure at a high school," *New England Journal of Medicine*, 342: 96–100 (January 13), 2000, p. 96.

21. S. Wessely, "Responding to mass psychogenic illness" (Editorial), *New England Journal of Medicine*, 342: 129–130 (January 13), 2000; p. 129.

22. Science writers make the same mistake. See L. K. Altman, "Mysterious illness often turns out to be mass hysteria," *New York Times*, January 18, 2000, Internet edition.

23. T. S. Szasz, *Pain and Pleasure.*

24. T. S. Szasz, *The Myth of Mental Illness.*

25. For the situation of the psychiatrist, see Chapter 5.

26. A. J. Barsky and J. F. Borus, "Functional somatic syndromes," *Annals of Internal Medicine*, 130: 910–921, 1999.

27. Ibid., p. 910.

28. Ibid.

29. See T. S. Szasz, *Pain and Pleasure.*

30. S. E. Ross, "*'Memes' as infectious agents in psychosomatic illness,*" *Annals of Internal Medicine*, 131: 867–871, 1999.

31. R. M. Berger, "What is psychopathology? And so what?" *Clinical Psychology*, 4: 235–248 (Fall), 1997; p. 245, emphasis added.

32. T. Duster, *Backdoor to Eugenics.* New York: Routledge, 1990, p. 69.

33. J. Leland, "Bad news in the bedroom," *Newsweek*, February 22, 1999, p. 47, emphasis added.

34. M. Bleuler, *The Schizophrenic Disorders*, p. 450.

35. For further discussion, see Chapter 4.

36. G. Kolata, "Using gene testing to decide a patient's treatment," *New York Times*, December 20, 1999, Internet edition.

37. G. B. Shaw, *The Intelligent Woman's Guide to Socialism, Capitalism, Sovietism and Fascism.* quoted in L. R. Frank, ed., *Random House Webster's Quotationary*, p. 521.

38. R. B. Fetter, "Background," in R. B. Fetter, ed., *DRGs*, pp. 3–47, p. 4.

39. E. Coiera, *Guide to Medical Informatics*, p. 162.

40. Ibid.

41. R. Levatter, "Economics 101 for doctors," *Vital Speeches of the Day*, 61: 590–595, 1995.

42. See Chapter 4 for further discussion.

43. American Psychiatric Association, "Introduction," *DSM-IV*, p. xxiii.

44. E. Coiera, *Guide to Medical Informatics*, p. xxi, emphasis added.

45. Ibid., p. 177.

46. I made this point more than forty years ago. See T. S. Szasz, "The classification of 'mental illness': A situational analysis of psychiatric operations," *Psychiatric Quarterly*, 33: 77–101 (January), 1959.

47. G. G. Gupta, "Diagnosis-related groups," *The Pharos*, Spring, 1990, pp. 12–17.

48. P. Klass, "Managing managed care," *New York Times Magazine*, October 5, 1997, p. 75, emphasis added.

49. Ibid., p. 74. In this connection, see J. Romains, *Knock.*

50. L. Lagnado, "Hospitals profit by 'upcoding' illnesses," *Wall Street Journal,* April 17, 1997, pp. B1 and B10; G. Anders, "Code confusion: Story of Jack Mills is lesson in the difficulty of policing Medicare," *Wall Street Journal* 1997, July 21, pp. A1 and A6.

51. A. Comarow, "Is your doctor lying for you? He probably is, and it's for your own good," *U.S. News & World Report,* October 25, 1999, pp. 60–61.

52. E. Rivera, "Dirty little diagnosis?" *Time,* February 7, 2000, p. 69. See also M. K. Wynia et al, "Physician manipulation of reimbursement rules for patients: Between a rock and a hard place," *JAMA,* 283:1858–1865 (April 12), 2000.

53. C. W. Smith, "90862: A code under siege," *Psychiatric Practice and Managed Care (APA),* 5: 3–5 (November–December) 1999, p. 3.

54. Ibid., p. 4.

55. J. Steinhauer, "Fraud case underscores debate for infertility care," *New York Times,* January 25, 2000, pp. 25, 29.

56. Ibid.

57. E. Rivera, "Dirty little diagnosis?" *Time,* February 7, 2000, p. 69.

58. J. Steinhauer, "Fraud case underscores debate for infertility care," *New York Times,* January 25, 2000, pp. 25, 29. Associated Press, "Fertility doctor jury deadlocks," *New York Times,* March 7, 2000, Internet edition.

59. V. G. Freeman, et al., "Lying for patients: Physician deception of third-party payers," *Archives of Internal Medicine,* 159: 2263–2270 (October 25), 1999. In this connection, see P. Zagorin, *Ways of Lying.*

60. T. S. Szasz, *Our Right to Drugs.*

61. V. G. Freeman et al., "Lying for patients: Physician deception of third-party payers," *Archives of Internal Medicine,* 159: 2263–2270 (October 25), 1999; and "Poll: Many doctors say it's ok to lie to insurers," *Sarasota (Florida) Herald-Tribune,* October 25, 1999, p. 1A.

62. Association News, "Medicare proposal could be dangerous, says DB head," *Psychiatric News,* 34: 4 (November 19), 1999.

63. Quoted in "Money," *Encyclopedia Britannica,* vol. 15, pp. 700–707, p. 700.

64. See C. Mackay, *Extraordinary Popular Delusions,* pp. 1–45.

65. Ibid., p. 703.

66. See Chapter 2.

67. J. Robitscher, *The Powers of Psychiatry,* p. 39; for a good semifictional account, see P. Barker, *Regeneration.*

68. C. W. Calomiris, "The impending collapse of the European Monetary Union," *Cato Journal,* 18: 445–452 (Winter), 1999.

69. R. A. Aronowitz, *Making Sense of Illness,* p. 187, emphasis added.

70. The pertinent literature is vast. See, for example, S. A. Kirk and H. Kutchins, *The Selling of DSM* and the references therein. For a recent example, see J. T. Bennett and T. J. DiLorenzo, *The Food and Drink Police.*

CHAPTER 4. CERTIFYING MEDICINE: DISABILITY

1. A. de Tocqueville, quoted in D. A. Stone, *The Disabled State,* p. 99.

2. W. Churchill, quoted in F. King, 'New Age hypochondria," *National Review*, March 29, 1993, p. 80.

3. H. H. Kessler, *Disability*, pp. 1, 25, emphasis added.

4. U.S. Department of Commerce, "Census brief," *CENBR/97–5,* December 1997.

5. Ibid.

6. Sutton vs. United Air Lines, 97–1943, 1999. L. Greenhouse, "High Court limits who is protected by disability law," *New York Times,* June 23, 1999, Internet edition.

7. T. S. Szasz, *The Manufacture of Madness.*

8. U.S. Department of Commerce, "Census brief," *CENBR/97–5,* December 1997.

9. See, for example, D. Grady, "A great pretender now faces the truth of illness," *New York Times,* July 20, 1999, Internet edition; and M. Feldman, C. C. Ford, and T. Reinhold, *Patient or Pretender.*

10. T. S. Szasz, *Cruel Compassion.*

11. G. Himmelfarb, *The Idea of Poverty.* See also T. S. Szasz, *Cruel Compassion,* Chapters 1, 2, and 5.

12. Quoted in D. A. Stone, *The Disabled State*, p. 79.

13. Ibid., p. 86, emphasis added.

14. Ibid., emphasis added.

15. Quoted in ibid., p. 80.

16. Ibid., pp. 82–83.

17. American Medical Association, *Guides to the Evaluation of Permanent Impairment*; and E. A. Spieler et al., "Recommendations to guide revision of the *Guides to the Evaluation of Permanent Impairment,*" *JAMA*, 283: 519–523 (January 26), 2000.

18. Ibid., p. 3.

19. Ibid., p. 87.

20. D. P. Phillips, N. Christenfeld, and N. M. Ryan, "An increase in the number of deaths in the United States in the first week of the month: An association with substance abuse and other causes of death," *New England Journal of Medicine*, 341: 93–98 (July 8), 1999, p. 93.

21. Ibid., pp. 93, 97.

22. N. Hellen and S. Farrar, "Hawking joins the celestial high earners," *Sunday Times* (London), March 28, 1999, p. 1/23.

23. Quoted in E. Walsh, "Strange love: The woman who wants to start a new life with John Hinckley, Jr.," *New Yorker*, April 5, 1999, pp. 51–67; pp. 54, 60.

24. J. D. Davidson, and W. Rees-Mogg, *The Great Reckoning*, p. 81.

25. See T. S. Szasz, *Cruel Compassion.*

26. D. A. Stone, *The Disabled State*, p. 58.

27. L. von Mises, *Socialism*, p. 432.

28. D. A. Stone, *The Disabled State*, p. 169.

29. J. Leo, "The new Trivial Pursuit," *U.S. News & World Report*, August 30, 1999, p. 20.

30. For detailed discussions of malingering, see T. S. Szasz, *The Myth of Mental Illness, Insanity,* and *The Untamed Tongue.*

31. T. Mann, *Confessions of Felix Krull.*

32. J. Gleick, *Genius.* See also V. Woolf, *On Being Ill.*

33. Plato, *Republic,* Paul Shorey translation in Plato, *The Collected Dialogues of Plato,* 405d, p. 844, emphasis added.

34. See, for example, T. S. Szasz, *Ideology and Insanity,* and "The sane slave: An historical note on the use of medical diagnosis as justificatory rhetoric," *American Journal of Psychotherapy,* 25: 228–239 (April), 1971.

35. O. von Bismarck, quoted in M. J. Lynch and S. S. Raphael, *Medicine and the State,* p. 15, emphasis added.

36. M. J. Lynch and S. S. Raphael, *Medicine and the State,* p. 36.

37. D. Smoot, "Socialized medicine" [1960], in Foundation for Economic Education, *Politicized Medicine,* pp. 123–126, p. 123.

38. See, for example, D. J. Rothman, "Medical professionalism—Focusing on the real issues," *New England Journal of Medicine,* 342: 1284–1286 (April 27), 2000; and J. Richmond and J. Eisenberg, "Medical professionalism in society," ibid., p. 1288.

39. M. J. Lynch and S. S. Raphael, *Medicine and the State,* p. 295.

40. Ibid., p. 296.

41. Ibid., p. 299.

42. E. Bleuler, *A Textbook of Psychiatry,* p. 191.

43. K. R. Eissler, "Malingering," in G. B. Wilbur and W. Muensterberger, eds., *Psychoanalysis and Culture,* pp. 252–253.

44. American Psychiatric Association, *Diagnostic and Statistical Manual of Mental Disorders-IV* (DSM-IV), p. 683.

45. Ibid., p. 471.

46. Ibid., p. 474.

47. P. Davis, "Principal fired for harassment draws disability: Technicality gives man $38,000-a-year Va. pension for 'psychosexual disorder,'" *Washington Post,* February 22, 1999. Internet edition, emphasis added.

48. J. Calderone, "Disabled teacher is skiing pro," *Daily News* (New York), February 22, 1999, Internet edition. For similar cases in Europe, see R. Scrutton, "In the Bulger case the justice system delivered a verdict which brought some peace to our troubled hearts, only to be subjected to mad Euro litigation," *Times* (London), March 16, 1999, Internet edition.

49. L. von Mises, *Human Action.* See also D. A. Stone, *The Disabled State,* especially Chapter 1; she recognizes only work-based and need-based distribution, and ignores crime (coercion) as a species of economic-social strategy for making a living.

50. See T. S. Szasz, *Cruel Compassion.*

51. See R. Raico, "Liberalism, Marxism, and the state," *The Cato Journal,* 11: 390–404 (Winter), 1992.

52. J. D. Davidson and W. Rees-Mogg, *The Great Reckoning,* p. 103.

53. M. Freudenheim, "New law to bring wider job rights for mentally ill," *New York Times,* September 23, 1991, pp. A1, D4.

54. M. J. Goldman, "Kleptomania: Making sense out of nonsense," *American Journal of Psychiatry*, 148: 986–996 (August), 1991.

55. In this connection, see M. Freedman, "How lawyers keep busy," *Forbes*, March 20, 2000, p. 92.

56. L. Greenhouse, "Act requires medical justification for institutionalization, Court says," *New York Times*, June 23, 1999, Internet edition.

57. T. S. Szasz, *Cruel Compassion*.

58. B. A. McLaughlin, "Myth of mental illness," *Canadian Underwriter*, 63: 36–40, March 1996.

59. Ibid., emphasis added.

60. H. H. Kessler, *Disability*, p. 233.

61. R. H. Haveman, V. Halberstadt, and R. V. Burkhauser, *Public Policy toward Disabled Workers*, p. 84.

62. J. F. Burton, Jr., "Workers' compensation, twenty-four-hour coverage, and managed care," in V. Reno, J. L. Mashaw, and B. Gradison, eds., *Disability*, p. 129.

63. R. H. Haveman, V. Halberstadt, and R. V. Burkhauser, *Public Policy toward Disabled Workers*, p. 84.

64. D. A. Stone, *The Disabled State*, pp. 9, 84.

65. Ibid., p. 168.

66. J. L. Mashaw, "Disability benefits policy: Is there a crisis?," in V. Reno, J. L. Mashaw, and B. Gradison, eds., *Disability*, p. 22.

67. B. C. Vladeck, E. O"Brien, T. Hoyer, and S. Clauser, "Challenges in Medicare and Medicaid for persons with disabilities," in ibid., p. 96.

68. M. Berkowitz, "Encouraging work through cash benefits policy: New proposals," in ibid., p. 50.

69. B. C. Vladeck, E. O'Brien, T. Hoyer, and S. Clauser, "Challenges in Medicare and Medicaid for Persons with Disabilities," in ibid., p. 87.

70. M. Topol, "Compensation case ruling opens door to psychiatric claims," *Newsday*, March 6, 2000, Internet edition, emphasis added.

71. R. H. Haveman, V. Halberstadt, and R. V. Burkhauser, *Public Policy toward Disabled Workers*, p. 462.

72. D. A. Stone, *The Disabled State*, p. 9, emphasis added.

73. Ibid., pp. 94–95, 96–97.

74. T. S. Szasz, *Cruel Compassion*.

CHAPTER 5. PSYCHIATRIC MEDICINE: DISORDER

1. M. Bleuler, *The Schizophrenic Disorders*, p. 448.

2. White House Press Office, "White House fact sheet on myths and facts about mental illness," June 5, 1999; "Myths and facts about mental illness," *New York Times*, June 7, 1999, Internet edition. See also, www.info@ariannaonline.com.

3. E. W. Campion, "Liberty and the control of tuberculosis" (Editorial), *New England Journal of Medicine*, 340: 385–386 (February 4), 1999.

4. American Psychiatric Association, "Introduction," *DSM-IV*, pp. xxi, xxv.

5. A. J. Frances, "Foreword," in J. Z. Sadler, O. P. Wigging, and M. A. Schwartz, eds., *Philosophical Perspectives on Psychiatric Diagnostic Classification,* pp. vii–ix, pp. vii–viii.

6. Ibid.

7. T. S. Szasz, *The Myth of Mental Illness, Insanity,* and *The Meaning of Mind.*

8. American Psychiatric Association, "Introduction," *DSM-IV,* p. xxii, emphasis added.

9. Ibid., p. xxiii.

10. Lilly, "1999 Annual Report," Indianapolis: Eli Lily and Company, 2000, pp. 14–15, emphasis added. See also www.lilly.com.

11. B. Rush, quoted in C. Binger, *Revolutionary Doctor,* p. 281.

12. R. Hunter and I. Macalpine, eds., *Three Hundred Years of Psychiatry,* p. 1027.

13. T. Meynert, *Psychiatry,* p. v, emphasis in the original.

14. W. Riese, "The neuropsychological phase in the history of psychiatric thought" in I. Galdston, *Historical Derivations of Modern Psychiatry,* pp. 75–137, p. 115. In this connection, see B. Libet, A. Freeman, and K. Sutherland, eds., "The volitional brain: Towards a neuroscience of free will," *Journal of Consciousness Studies,* vol. 6, issue 8–9, August-September 1999, Internet edition: www.imprint.co.uk.

15. S. Freud, "An autobiographical study" [1924], in *SE,* vol. 20, pp. 1–76, p. 12.

16. T. S. Szasz, *The Myth of Mental Illness.*

17. R. Hunter, "Some lessons from the history of psychiatry" (Abstract), *Society for the Social History of Medicine Bulletin,* 5: 11–12, 1971; quoted in M. S. Micale, and R. Porter, eds., *Discovering the History of Psychiatry,* pp. 83–94, p. 90, emphasis added.

18. R. Hunter and I. Macalpine, *Psychiatry for the Poor, 1851,* pp. 11–12, emphasis added.

19. N. C. Andreasen, "What is psychiatry?", *American Journal of Psychiatry,* 154: 591– 593 (May), 1997.

20. S. B. Guze, "Biological psychiatry: Is there any other kind?," *Psychological Medicine,* 19: 315–323, 1989, emphasis in the original.

21. D. F. Klein and P. H. Wender, *Understanding Depression,* p. 4, emphasis added.

22. T. S. Szasz, *The Myth of Mental Illness, Schizophrenia,* and *The Meaning of Mind.*

23. E. von Feuchtersleben, *Medical Psychology,* quoted in D. Schreber, *Memoirs,* p. 412.

24. E. Kraepelin, *Lectures on Clinical Psychiatry* and *Einführung in die psychiatrische Klinik,* p. 1, emphasis added.

25. E. Bleuler, *Dementia Praecox or the Group of Schizophrenias,* pp. 279, 327, emphasis added.

26. J. F. Kennedy, "Message from the President of the United States relative to mental illness and mental retardation," February 5, 1963, 88th Congress, 1st session. H. Rep. Document No. 58.

27. Quoted in Office of the Press Secretary of the President of the United States, "Remarks by the President, the First Lady, the Vice President, and Mrs. Gore at White House Conference on Mental Health," Blackburn Auditorium, Howard University, Washington, DC, June 7, 1999. Arianna Online, 1158 26th Street, Suite #428, Santa Monica, CA 90403, E-mail: info@ariannaonline.com.

28. Ibid., emphasis added.

29. H. R. Clinton, *It Takes a Village*, p. 64, and Office of the Press Secretary, The White House, "Remarks by the President, the First Lady, The Vice President, and Mrs. Gore, at White House Conference on Mental Health," Blackburn Auditorium, Howard University, Washington, DC, June 7, 1999, Internet edition.

30. D. Satcher, quoted in "Satcher discusses MH issues hurting black community," *Psychiatric News*, 34: 6 (October 15), 1999, emphasis added.

31. For further discussion, see Chapter 7.

32. L. Tolstoy, *Anna Karenina*, in J. Bartlett, *Familiar Quotations*, 12th edition, p. 1192.

33. J. L. Levenson, "Psychiatric commitment and involuntary hospitalization: An ethical perspective," *Psychiatric Quarterly*, 58: 106–112 (Summer), 1986–1987; p. 106, emphasis added. See also P. Chodoff, "Involuntary hospitalization of the mentally ill as a moral issue," *American Journal of Psychiatry*, 141: 384–389, 1984.

34. T. S. Szasz, *Insanity, and Cruel Compassion.*

35. "Public health law," in *McKinney's Consolidated Laws of New York*, Book 44; Public Health Law, Articles 2200–2270, Control of Tuberculosis, pp. 52–73; Control of Sexually Transmitted Diseases, Articles 2300–2311, pp. 74–90.

36. M. R. Gasner, et al., "The use of legal action in New York City to ensure treatment of tuberculosis," *New England Journal of Medicine*, 340: 359–366 (February 4), 1999.

37. K. Neal, "Compulsory treatment for infectious disease" (Letter), *The Lancet*, 343: 675 (March 12), 1994, emphasis added.

38. M. Morton and R. Marshall, "Public interest versus confidentiality in notifiable diseases" (Letter), *The Lancet*, 343: 359 (February 5), 1994.

39. E. F. Torrey and J. Miller, "Can psychiatry learn from tuberculosis treatment?" *Psychiatric Services*, 50: 1389 (November), 1999, emphasis added.

40. H. Minkoff and N. Santoro, "Ethical considerations in the treatment of infertility in women with human immunodeficiency virus infection," *New England Journal of Medicine*, 342: 1748–1750 (June 8), 2000.

41. Quoted in R. Dewey, "The jury law for commitment of the insane in Illinois (1867–1893), and Mrs. E. P. W. Packard, its author, also later developments in lunacy legislation in Illinois," *American Journal of Insanity*, 69: 571–584 (January), 1913, emphasis added. For details, see T. S. Szasz, *The Manufacture of Madness.*

42. *Kansas v. Leroy Hendricks, No. 95–1649,* "Excerpts from opinions on status of sex offenders," *New York Times*, June 24, 1997, p. B11.

43. Associated Press, "Jury: 95–year-old sexual predator is still a threat," *Syracuse Herald-Journal,* February 2, 2000, p. A8, emphasis added.

44. D. J. Jaffe, "How to prepare for an emergency," (2000), http://www.nami. org/about/naminyc/coping/911.html. More than half a century ago, James Thurber parodied the commitment process in his short essay "The unicorn in the garden," reprinted in T. S. Szasz, ed., *The Age of Madness,* pp. 278–279.

45. T. S. Szasz, *The Myth of Mental Illness.*

46. S. Arieti, *Interpretation of Schizophrenia,* p. 4, emphasis added.

47. L. Reznek, *The Philosophical Defence of Psychiatry,* pp. 204, 213.

48. R. E. Kendell, "The concept of disease and its implications for psychiatry" [1975], in A. L. Caplan, H. T. Engelhardt, Jr., and J. J. McCartney, eds., *Concepts of Health and Disease,* pp. 443–458, p. 449.

49. G. L. Engel, "The need for a new medical model: A challenge to biomedicine," in A. L. Caplan, H. T. Engelhardt, Jr., and J. J. McCartney, eds., *Concepts of Health and Disease,* pp. 589– 607, p. 599, emphasis added.

50. Ibid., p. 595.

51. D. W. Goodwin, and S. B. Guze, *Psychiatric Diagnosis,* p. xi, emphasis added.

52. For example, see A. Frances in, "APA Board accepts new diagnostic manual for mental illness," *The Bulletin* (New York State Psychiatric Association), 36: 9, 11 (September/October) 1993.

53. H. T. Engelhardt, Jr., "The concepts of health and disease," in A. L. Caplan, H. T. Engelhardt, Jr., J. J. and McCartney, eds., *Concepts of Health and Disease,* pp. 31–45, p. 32.

54. Ibid., pp. 37, 41.

55. C. Rycroft, *A Critical Dictionary of Psychoanalysis,* p. 102, emphasis added.

56. J. Wakefield, "The concept of mental disorder: On the boundary between biological facts and social values," *American Psychologist,* 47: 373–388, 1992.

57. R. M. Berger, "What is psychopathology? And so what?" *Clinical Psychology,* 4: 235–248 (Fall), 1997, p. 235.

58. Ibid., pp. 245–246.

59. See Chapter 3 on the relationship between disease and disability.

60. P. E. Nathan, "In the final analysis, it's the data that count," *Clinical Psychology,* 4: 281–284 (Fall), 1997, p. 281.

61. K. Menninger, *The Crime of Punishment,* p. 77.

62. L. J. Duhl, "Confessions of a psychotherapist," *Bulletin of the Menninger Clinic,* 63: 538–546 (Fall), 1999, p. 540.

63. For example, see J. Gibeaut, "Who knows best? It's an ongoing debate: Should the government force treatment on the mentally ill?" *ABA (American Bar Association) Journal,* January 2000. http://www.abanet.org/journal.

64. C. Thomas, "Dissenting opinion," in *Foucha v. Louisiana,* 563 So. 2d 1138, reversed. No. 90–5844, decided May 18, 1992.

65. T. S. Szasz, "Parity for mental illness, disparity for the mental patient," *The Lancet,* 352: 1213–1215 (October 10), 1998.

66. Associated Press, "Psychiatric hospital accused of holding patients captive in Fla.," *Arizona Republic,* December 14, 1996, p. A9.

67. G. K. Chesterton, *Orthodoxy,* p. 32.

68. R. de. Sousa, "The politics of mental illness," *Inquiry,* 15: 187–202, 1972, p. 201.

69. Aristotle, *Poetics,* 1459a, in *The Basic Works of Aristotle,* p. 1479.

70. R. E. Kendell, "Schizophrenia: A Medical View of a Medical Concept," in W. F. Flack, Jr., D. R. Miller, and M. Wiener, eds. *What is Schizophrenia?,* pp. 9–72, p. 60.

71. See, for example, "Medical device fights female impotence," *USA Today,* May 4, 2000, p. 8D.

72. S. A. Cartwright, "Report on the diseases and physical peculiarities of the Negro race," *New Orleans Medical and Surgical Journal,* 7: 691–715, 1851; and T. S. Szasz, "The sane slave: An historical note on the use of medical diagnosis as justificatory rhetoric," *American Journal of Psychotherapy,* 25: 228–239 (April), 1971.

73. See T. S. Szasz, *The Manufacture of Madness.*

74. R. Krafft-Ebing, *Psychopathia Sexualis,* pp. vi, vii, emphasis added.

75. Ibid., pp. 52–54.

76. S. Freud, *The Psychopathology of Everyday Life,* in *SE,* vol. 6.

77. S. Freud, *The Complete Letters of Sigmund Freud to Wilhelm Fliess,* p. 345.

78. Ibid., p. 40.

79. Ibid., p. 41.

80. Ibid., p. 50.

81. Ibid., p. 94.

82. Ibid., p. 98.

83. Ibid., p. 287.

84. Ibid., p. 380.

85. I. W. Charny, "Genocide and mass destruction: Doing harm to others as a missing dimension of psychopathology," *Psychiatry,* 49:144–157 (May), 1986, p. 144, emphasis added.

86. A. Poussaint, quoted in "Is extreme racism a mental illness?," *The New Crisis,* January–February, 2000, pp. 23–25, p. 23, emphasis added; see also "They hate. They kill. Are they insane?," *New York Times,* August 26, 1999, Internet edition.

87. T. S. Szasz, *The Manufacture of Madness, Ideology and Insanity, Psychiatric Justice, Psychiatric Slavery, Cruel Compassion.*

88. See T. S. Szasz, "Patriotic poisoners," *Humanist,* 36: 5–7 (November–December), 1976; J. Marks, *The Search for the "Manchurian Candidate."*

89. B. H. Price, R. D. Adams, and J. T. Coyle, "Neurology and psychiatry: Closing the great divide," *Neurology,* 54: 8–14 (January), 2000, pp. 10–11, emphasis added.

90. See J. A. Schaler, *Addiction is a Choice.*

91. See, for example, D. Bookchin and J. Schumacher, "The virus and the vaccine," *The Atlantic Monthly,* February 2000, pp. 68–80.

92. G. S. Stent, "Molecular biology and metaphysics," *Nature,* 248: 779–781 (April 26), 1974. For a typical popular example, see the cover story "Why we fall in

love: Biology, not romance, guides Cupid's arrow," *U.S. News & World Report*, February 7, 2000, pp. 42–48.

93. B. H. Price, R. D. Adams, and J. T. Coyle, "Neurology and psychiatry: Closing the great divide," *Neurology*, 54: 8–14 (January), 2000, pp. 12–13.

94. J. Gibeaut, "Who knows best? It's an ongoing debate: Should the government force treatment on the mentally ill?" *ABA (American Bar Association) Journal*, January 2000, http://www.abanet.org/journal, emphasis added.

95. Ibid., emphasis added.

96. W. Shakespeare, *A Midsummer Night's Dream*, Act 5, scene 1, lines 15–17.

97. Quoted in S. L. Gilman, "The image of the hysteric," in S. L. Gilman, H. King, R. Porter, G. S. Rousseau, and E. Showalter, *Hysteria beyond Freud*, pp. 345–452, p. 436.

98. K. Woodward, *Making Saints,* pp. 15, 17.

99. Ibid., p. 17.

100. Ibid., p. 19.

101. Associated Press, "Catholics in Mexico celebrate 27 new saints," *Syracuse Herald-American,* May 21, 2000, p. A2.

102. K. Woodward, *Making Saints,* pp. 374–375.

103. Ibid., p. 380, emphasis in the original.

104. See, for example, P. Landesman, "A 20th-century master scam," *New York Times Magazine,* July 18, 1999, pp. 31–64. See also M. Jones, ed., *Fake?* and T. S. Szasz, *The Myth of Mental Illness.*

105. P. Gourevitch, "The memory thief," *New Yorker*, June 14, 1999, pp. 49–66.

106. T. S. Szasz, *The Myth of Mental Illness.*

107. J. P. Sloan, *Jerzy Kosinski*, p. 223.

108. C. Ozick, "Holocaust literature" (Letters), *Commentary*, June 1999, pp. 6–8, p. 7.

109. B. Wilkomirski, *Fragments.*

110. Quoted in P. Gourevitch, "The memory thief," *New Yorker*, June 14, 1999, pp. 49– 66, p. 50.

111. Quoted in ibid.

112. C. Ozick, "Holocaust literature" (Letters), *Commentary*, June 1999, pp. 6–8, p. 7, emphasis added.

113. R. Pear, "Mental disorders common, U.S. says: Many not treated," *New York Times*, December 13, Internet edition.

114. D. Shalala, "Message from Donna E. Shalala," in "Mental Health: A Report of the Surgeon General," December 14, 1999, http://www.surgeongeneral.gov/library/mental health.

115. Quoted in R. Pear, "Mental disorders common, U.S. says: Many not treated," *New York Times*, December 13, Internet edition.

116. M. Astell, *The Christian Religion, as Profess'd by a Daughter of the Church of England*, 1705, p. 95, quoted in G. S. Rousseau, ed., *The Languages of Psyche*, p. xvii, emphasis in the original.

CHAPTER 6. PHILOSOPHICAL MEDICINE: CRITIQUE OR RATIFICATION?

1. E. Burke, "Jacobinism," in L. I. Bredvold and R. G. Ross, eds., *The Philosophy of Edmund Burke*, p. 249.

2. H. Greenberg, "Introductory Remarks: Medicine Took an Earlier Flight," in P. R. Gross, N. Levitt, and M. W. Lewis, *The Flight from Science and Reason*, pp. ix-xi, p. ix.

3. G. Hesslow, "Do we need a concept of disease?" *Theoretical Medicine*, 14: 1–14, 1993, p. 3.

4. K. W. M. Fulford, *Moral Theory and Medical Practice*, p. 275.

5. G. Khushf, "Why bioethics needs the philosophy of medicine," *Theoretical Medicine*, 18: 145–163, 1997, p. 159.

6. See S. Bloch, P. Chodoff, and S. A. Green, eds., *Psychiatric Ethics*.

7. R. Virchow, "Concerning standpoints in scientific medicine" (1847), in A. L. Caplan, H. T. Engelhardt, Jr., and J. J. McCartney, eds., *Concepts of Health and Disease*, pp. 188–190, p. 188, emphasis added.

8. M. J. Adler, *What Man Has Made of Man*, p. 204.

9. P. Sedgwick, "Illness—mental and otherwise,"in A. L. Caplan, H. T. Engelhardt, Jr., and J. J. McCartney, eds., *Concepts of Health and Disease*, pp. 119–129, pp. 120–121.

10. Ibid., emphasis in the original.

11. Ibid., pp. 123, 127, emphasis in the original.

12. R. A. Aronowitz, *Making Sense of Illness*, p. 7.

13. C. Boorse, "On the distinction between disease and illness" (1975), in T. L. Beauchamp and L. Walters, eds., *Contemporary Issues in Bioethics*, pp. 120–131, quoting I. Gregory, *Fundamental of Psychiatry*, p. 32.

14. Ibid., p. 128.

15. H. Fabrega, Jr., "The scientific usefulness of the idea of illness," in A. L. Caplan, H. T. Engelhardt, Jr., and J. J. McCartney, eds., *Concepts of Health and Disease*, pp. 131–142, p. 131.

16. Ibid., pp. 134, 135, emphasis added.

17. A. Kleinman, *The Illness Narratives*, p. 5.

18. L. Eisenberg, "Disease and illness: Distinctions between professional and popular ideas of sickness," *Culture, Medicine, and Psychiatry*, 1: 9–23, 1977, p. 11.

19. Ibid., p. 9, emphasis added.

20. T. S. Szasz, *Law, Liberty, and Psychiatry* and *Anti-Freud*.

21. K. W. M. Fulford, *Moral Theory and Medical Practice*, p. 28, emphasis added.

22. Ibid., p. 146, emphasis added.

23. K. W. M. Fulford, "Closet logics: Hidden conceptual elements in the DSM and ICF classifications of mental disorders," in J. Z. Sadler, 0. P. Wiggins, and M. A. Schwartz, eds., *Philosophical Perspectives on Psychiatric Diagnostic Classification*, pp. 211– 232, pp. 211–212, emphasis added.

24. K. W. M. Fulford, *Moral Theory and Medical Practice*, pp. 76, 149, emphasis added.

25. A. Fadiman, *The Spirit Catches You and You Fall Down*, p. 95.

26. K. W. M. Fulford, *Moral Theory and Medical Practice*, p. 188.

27. See T. S. Szasz, *Fatal Freedom*.

28. M. Warnock, "Philosophical foreword," in K. W. M. Fulford, *Moral Theory and Medical Practice*, pp. vii–ix, pp. vii–viii.

29. Ibid., p. viii.

30. Ibid.

31. Ibid., p. viii.

32. R. L. Woolfolk, "Malfunction and mental illness," *Monist*, 82: 658–671 (October), 1999, p. 670.

33. C. M. Culver and B. Gert, *Philosophy in Medicine*, p. 3.

34. Ibid., p. 4.

35. Ibid., p. 67.

36. Ibid., p. vii.

37. Ibid., p. 81, emphasis in the original.

38. Ibid., p. 95. The authors cite G. Engel, "Is grief a disease?" *Psychosomatic Medicine*, 23: 18–22, 1961, emphasis added.

39. C. M. Culver and B. Gert, *Philosophy in Medicine*, pp. 65, 91, emphasis added.

40. B. Gert, C. M. Culver, and K. D. Clouser, *Bioethics*, pp. 98–119, emphasis added.

41. C. M. Culver and B. Gert, *Philosophy in Medicine*, p. 22.

42. Ibid., p. 165.

43. R. Hare, "The philosophical basis of medical ethics," in S. Bloch and P. Chodoff, eds., *Psychiatric Ethics*, pp. 33–46, p. 42, emphasis in the original.

44. T. S. Szasz, *Fatal Freedom*, especially Chapter 4.

45. R. Miller, "The ethics of involuntary commitment to mental health treatment," in S. Bloch and P. Chodoff, eds., *Psychiatric Ethics*, pp. 265–289, p. 268.

46. Ibid., emphasis added.

47. P. Kurtz, "The growth of antiscience," *Skeptical Inquirer*, 18: 255–267 (Spring), 1994.

48. R. Porter, "The body and the mind, the doctor and the patient: Negotiating hysteria," in S. L. Gilman, H. King, R. Porter, G. S. Rousseau, and E. Showalter, *Hysteria beyond Freud*, pp. 225–285, pp. 233–234, emphasis added.

49. Ibid., p. 234.

50. R. Dixon, *The Baumgarten Corruption*, p. 115, pp. 153–154.

51. Quoted in Lifeline, "Kennedy Shortridge," *The Lancet*, 355: 328 (January 22), 2000.

52. G. W. Geelhoed, "Metabolic maladaptation: Individual and social consequences of medical intervention in correcting endemic hypothyroidism," *Nutrition*, 15: 908–932, 1999.

53. G. W. Geelhoed, "An author's editorial: Health care advocacy in world health," *Nutrition,* 15: 940–943, 1999, p. 942.

54. J. Sugarman, "Moral maladaptation? Reflections on a report on research involving the correction of endemic hypothyroidism in Africa," *Nutrition,* 15: 934–935, 1999, p. 935, emphasis added.

55. C. S. Lewis, "The humanitarian theory of punishment" [1953], in C. S. Lewis, *God in the Dock,* pp. 287–294, pp. 292–293.

56. Quoted in Office of the Press Secretary of the President of the United States, "Remarks by the President, the First Lady, the Vice President, and Mrs. Gore at White House Conference on Mental Health," Blackburn Auditorium, Howard University, Washington, DC, June 7, 1999. Arianna Online, 1158 26th Street, Suite #428, Santa Monica, CA 90403, E-mail: info@ariannaonline.com.

57. A. Quindlen, "The C word in the hallways," *Newsweek,* November 29, 1999, p. 112.

58. Quoted in O. Chadwick, *Professor Lord Acton,* p. xii.

CHAPTER 7. POLITICAL MEDICINE: THE
THERAPEUTIC STATE

1. Quoted in B. D. Porter, *War and the Rise of the State,* p. 10.

2. R. Bourne, *The Radical Will,* p. 360.

3. State of Colorado, Second Regular Session, Sixty-second General Assembly, "A bill for an act concerning the policy of addressing the disease of obesity in a medically appropriate manner," www.state.co.us/gov_dir/stateleg.htlm, February 2000. The bill did not pass.

4. S. Woloshin and L. M. Schwartz, "The U.S. Postal Service and cancer screening—stamps of approval?" *New England Journal of Medicine,* 340: 884–887 (March 18), 1999.

5. F. M. Watkins, "State: The concept," in *International Encyclopedia of the Social Sciences,* edited by D. L. Sills, vol. 15, pp. 150–157, p. 150; F. H. Fried, "State: The institution," in ibid., vol. 15, pp. 143–150, pp. 143, 149.

6. T. S. Szasz, *Law, Liberty, and Psychiatry,* p. 212.

7. See T. S. Szasz, "Toward the therapeutic state," *New Republic,* December 11, 1965, pp. 26–29; "Justice in the therapeutic state" [1970], in *The Theology of Medicine,* pp. 118–133; "Therapeutic tyranny," *Omni,* March 1980, p. 43; "Building the therapeutic state," *Contemporary Psychology,* 27: 297 (April), 1982; *The Therapeutic State* (1984); "The therapeutic state is a modern Leviathan," *Wall Street Journal Europe,* January 11, 1994, p. 9; "Diagnosis in the therapeutic state," *Liberty,* 7: 25–28 (September), 1994; "Idleness and lawlessness in the therapeutic state," *Society,* 32: 30–35 (May/June), 1995; "Routine neonatal circumcision: Symbol of the birth of the therapeutic state," *Journal of Medicine and Philosophy,* 21: 137–148, 1996.

8. G. Washington, quoted in *CATO Newsletter,* CATO Institute, June 1, 2000, p. 1.

9. E. P. Richards and K. C. Rathbun, ""The role of the police power in 21st century public health," *Sexually Transmitted Diseases*, 26: 350–357 (July) 1999; p. 356.

10. Ibid., emphasis added.

11. D. E. Beauchamp, *The Health of the Republic*, p. 136.

12. R. Virchow, "Scientific method and therapeutic standpoints" [1849], in L. J. Rather, ed., *Disease, Life, and Man*, pp. 40–66, p. 66, emphasis added.

13. Ibid., emphasis added.

14. See Chapters 3 and 5.

15. Quoted in B. D. Porter, *War and the Rise of the State*, p. xiii.

16. Quoted in W. F. Buckley, Jr., "The pursuit of AIDS in Africa," *National Review*, June 5, 2000, pp. 62–63.

17. See J. T. Flynn, *The Roosevelt Myth*.

18. Quoted in R. Higgs, *Crisis and Leviathan*, p. 159.

19. G. J. Danton, quoted in *Bartlett's Familiar Quotations*, edited by Justin Kaplan, 16th ed., p. 364.

20. George Jacques Danton, *Encyclopaedia Britannica*, vol. 7, p. 64.

21. R. Higgs, *Crisis and Leviathan.*, p. x.

22. M. van Creveld, *The Rise and Decline of the State*, p. vii.

23. See also N. Lawson, *The Retreat of the State*; S. Strange, *The Retreat of the State;* and D. Swann, *The Retreat of the State*. The title seems to have caught on.

24. R. J. Samuelson, "Who governs?" *Newsweek*, February 21, 2000, p. 33.

25. "1993 appropriations for National Institutes of Health," *Chronicle of Higher Education,* October 14, 1992, p. A-27.

26. J. Sharkey, *Bedlam*, p. 240.

27. J. Sharkey, "Mental illness hits the money trail," *New York Times,* June 6, 1999, Internet edition.

28. J. L. Nolan, Jr., *The Therapeutic State*, pp. 7–8; and J. D. Hogan, "International psychology in the next century: Comment and speculation from a U.S. perspective," *World Psychology*, 1: 9–25 (January), 1995.

29. U.S. Department of Health and Human Services, *Health, United States, 1998*, pp. 341–342.

30. Ibid., p. 345.

31. *World Almanac*, pp. 108–109.

32. J. M. Buchanan, *The Limits of Liberty*, p. 162.

33. T. S. Szasz, *Cruel Compassion*, especially pp. 150–186.

34. J. Gibeaut, "Who knows best? It's an ongoing debate: Should the government force treatment on the mentally ill?" *ABA (American Bar Association) Journal*, January 2000, http://www.abanet.org/journal.

35. B. D. Porter, *War and the Rise of the State*, p. 9, emphasis added.

36. D. E. Beauchamp "Community: The neglected tradition of public health," in D. E. Beauchamp and B. Steinbock, eds., *New Ethics for the Public's Health*, pp. 57–67, p. 59.

37. B. Streisand, "Network noodling: Who controls content?" *U.S. News & World Report*, January 24, 2000, p. 26.

38. D. Forbes, "Washington script doctors: How the government rewrote an episode of the WB's 'Smart Guy,' " *Salon*, January 13, 2000; M. Frankel, "Plots for hire: Media mercenaries join the war on drugs," *New York Times Magazine*, February 6, 2000, pp. 32–33.

39. B. Streisand, "Network noodling: Who controls content?" *U.S. News & World Report*, January 24, 2000, p. 26.

40. F. Morgan, "Is the White House involved in prime-time propaganda?" *Salon*, January 15, 2000.

41. R. D. Bonnette, "Anti-drug TV scripts," *New York Times*, January 18, 2000, p. A26.

42. G. Rose, "Sick individuals and sick populations," *International Journal of Epidemiology*, 14: 32–38, 1985; reprinted in D. E. Beauchamp, and B. Steinbock, eds., *New Ethics for the Public's Health*, pp. 28–38, pp. 36–37.

43. G. Dworkin, "Paternalism" (1972), in D. E. Beauchamp and B. Steinbock, eds., *New Ethics for the Public's Health*, pp. 115–128; pp. 127–128.

44. F. Germer, "The helmet issue—again," *U.S. News & World Report*, June 19, 2000, p. 30.

45. W. F. Stone, Jr., "State's power to require an individual to protect himself," *Washington and Lee Law Review*, 26: 112–119, 1969; p. 112.

46. Ibid., pp. 113–114.

47. Ibid., p. 114.

48. Quoted in D. Samuels, "Saying yes to drugs," *New Yorker*, March 23, 1998, pp. 48–55, pp. 48–49.

49. W. Gaylin and B. Jennings, *The Perversion of Autonomy*.

50. Quoted in R. Dubos, *Pasteur*, p. 307.

51. A. I. Leshner, "Science-based views of drug addiction and its treatment," *JAMA*, 282: 1314–1316 (October 13), 1999.

52. S. Satel, "For addicts, force is the best medicine," *Wall Street Journal*, January 7, 1998, p. 6.

53. Ibid.

54. K. E. Finkelstein, "New York to offer most addicts treatment instead of jail terms," *New York Times*, June 23, 2000, Internet edition; and Associated Press, "Plan for nonviolent addicts coming," ibid., emphasis added.

55. J. S. Kaye, "My turn: Making the case for hands-on courts," *Newsweek*, October 11, 1999, p. 13.

56. See Associated Press, "Fat man is told: To jail or shape up," *New York Times*, August 27, 1995, p. 12; Associated Press, "Internet-addicted mom loses custody of kids," *Syracuse Herald-Journal*, March 22, 1998.

57. J. L. Nolan, Jr., *The Therapeutic State*, pp. 97, 99.

58. "MH courts said to keep mentally ill out of jail," *Psychiatric News*, 34: 10 (November 5), 1999; S. E. Christian, "Special court for mentally ill in talking stage," *Chicago Tribune*, November 7, 1999, p. A13, emphasis added.

59. C. E. Koop and G. D. Lundberg, "Violence in America: A public health emergency" (Editorial), *JAMA*, 267: 3076 (June 10), 1992.

60. L. H. Ferry, L. M. Grissino, and P. S. Runfola, "Tobacco dependence curriculum in US undergraduate medical education," *JAMA*, 282: 825–828 (September 1), 1999.

61. P. J. Cook, et al., "The medical costs of gunshot injuries in the United States," *JAMA*, 282: 447–454 (August 4), 1999.

62. G. J. Wintemute, "The future of firearm violence prevention," *JAMA*, 282: 475–478 (August 4), 1999.

63. V. Iacopino and R. J. Waldman, "War and health: From Solferino to Kosovo—the evolving role of the physician," *JAMA*, 282: 475–478 (August 4), 1999.

64. T. B. Cole and A. Flanagin, "What can we do about violence?" *JAMA*, 282: 481– 482 (August 4), 1999.

65. M. Phillips, "Tyranny of the new body snatchers," *Sunday Times* (London), July 11, 1999, p. 1/17.

66. Quoted in "Notable & Quotable," *Wall Street Journal,* July 30, 1999, p. A14.

67. Quoted in F. MacCarthy, "Skin deep," *New York Review of Books*, October 7, 1999, pp. 19–20; p. 19.

68. S. Bevan and M. Prescott, "Blair launches personal carers to save family," *Sunday Times* (London), September 27, 1999, Internet edition.

69. *The Oxford Dictionary of Quotations,* p. 234.

70. S. Webb and B. Webb, *The State and the Doctor*, p. 1.

71. Ibid., p. 238, emphasis added.

72. Ibid., p. 239, emphasis added.

73. R. N. Proctor, *The Nazi War on Cancer*, p. 74.

74. See T. S. Szasz, *The Manufacture of Madness* and *The Therapeutic State*, especially pp. 213–238; also S. Bloch and P. Reddaway, *Psychiatric Terror*.

75. I. Kershaw, *Hitler,* p. 494.

76. Ibid., p. 541.

77. S. L. Gilman, "The Image of the Hysteric," in S. L. Gilman, H. King, R. Porter, G. S. Rousseau, and E. Showalter, *Hysteria beyond Freud*, pp. 345–452, p. 435.

78. S. Sontag, "America," *Partisan Review*, Winter, 1967, pp. 51–58, pp. 57–58.

79. P. Weindling, *Health, Race and German Politics between National Unification and Nazism, 1870–1945*, p. 1.

80. Ibid., pp. 2, 6.

81. Ibid., p. 14.

82. Ibid., pp. 7, 19.

83. Ibid., p. 283.

84. Ibid., p. 525.

85. Ibid., p. 518.

86. Ibid., pp. 544, 549.

87. Ibid., p. 550.

88. Ibid., pp. 576–577, 542–543.

89. Ibid., p. 537.

90. R. N. Proctor, *The Nazi War on Cancer*, p. 277.

91. H. Friedlander, *The Origin of Nazi Genocide*, pp. 180–181.

92. R. N. Proctor, *The Nazi War on Cancer*, p. 252.

93. Ibid., p. 11, emphasis added.

94. Ibid., p. 120.

95. Ibid., p. 58.

96. Ibid., p. 26.

97. Ibid., p. 136.

98. Ibid., p. 129, and J. Borkin, *The Crime and Punishment of I. G. Farben*, p. 58.

99. P. Singer, *Practical Ethics* and *Rethinking Life and Death.* See also "Dangerous words," *Princeton Alumni Weekly*, January 26, 2000, pp. 18–19; T. S. Szasz, *Fatal Freedom*, pp. 89, 96–97.

100. R. N. Proctor, *The Nazi War on Cancer*, p. 249, emphasis added.

101. Ibid., p. 271.

102. T. Jefferson, "Primary care physicians and posttraumatic stress disorder," *JAMA*, vol. 282, November 10, 1999, Internet edition.

103. N. Labi, "The grief brigade," *Time*, May 17, 1999, p. 69; D. Seligman, "Good grief! The counselors are everywhere!" *Forbes,* March 20, 2000, pp. 122–124. The situation in Britain is similar; see K. Toolis, "Shock tactics," *The Guardian Weekend* (UK), November 13, 1999, pp. 27–35.

104. B. D. Porter, *War and the Rise of the State*, p. 200.

105. W. H. Auden, *The Dyer's Hand, and Other Essays,* p. 14.

106. *DSM-IV*, p. 424.

107. Quoted in T. Jefferson, "Primary care physicians and posttraumatic stress disorder," *JAMA*, vol. 282, November 10, 1999, Internet edition.

108. Ibid., emphasis added.

109. J. Acocella, "Burned again," *New Yorker,* November 15, 1999, p. 98.

110. "Residents need support after patient suicide," *Psychiatric News*, 34: 24 (November 5), 1999.

111. T. S. Szasz, *Fatal Freedom.*

112. B. R. Bloom, "The wrong rights: We need rights to prevention, not just treatment," *Newsweek*, October 11, 1999, p. 92, emphasis added.

113. "Psychiatry in 21st century requires shift in public health model," *Psychiatric News,* 34: 25, 43 (October 1), 1999; p. 25.

114. D. Satcher, "The framework Convention on tobacco control: A report from the 52nd World Health Assembly," *JAMA*, 282: 424 (August 4), 1999.

115. Associated Press, "Surgeon general seeks effort to halt epidemic of suicide," *Washington Times*, September 29, 1999, Internet edition, emphasis added.

116. Ibid, emphasis added.

117. K. J. Arrow, "Uncertainty and the welfare economics of medical care," *American Economic Review*, 53: 941–973 (December) 1963, p. 967; see also E. Gahr, "Psyched out in left field," *American Spectator*, November 1999, pp. 66–67.

118. Office of the Press Secretary, The White House, "The Clinton Administration unveils initiative to protect consumers buying prescription drug products over the Internet," December 28, 1999, http://www.whitehouse.gov/library/this week, December 30, 1999, emphasis added.

119. See J. Bovard, *Freedom in Chains.*

120. Quoted in ibid., p. 15.

121. Quoted in ibid.

122. Quoted in ibid., p. 55, emphasis added.

123. Quoted in ibid.

124. A. Meiklejohn, *Political Freedom,* p. 13.

125. Quoted in J. Bovard, *Freedom in Chains,* p. 51.

126. D. E. Beauchamp, *Health Care Reform,* p. 113, emphasis added.

127. Ibid., p. 38.

128. D. E. Beauchamp, *The Health of the Republic,* p. ix.

129. Ibid., pp. 3, 8, emphasis added.

130. D. E. Beauchamp, "Public health as social justice," in D. E. Beauchamp and B. Steinbock, eds., *New Ethics for the Public's Health,* pp. 101–109, p. 109.

131. D. E. Beauchamp, *The Health of the Republic,* pp. 51, 150.

132. Ibid., p. 40.

133. Ibid., p. 155, emphasis in the original.

134. Ibid., p. 156.

135. H. Waitzkin, *The Second Sickness,* p. 7.

136. Ibid., pp. 67–68.

137. Ibid., p. 211.

138. Ibid., p. 224.

139. L. Eisenberg, "Whatever happened to the faculty on the way to the agora?" *Archives of Internal Medicine,* 159: 2251–2256 (October 25), 1999. For the realities of universal health insurance, see, for example, L. Rogers and C. Dignan, "NHS patients cross Channel to jump queues," *Sunday Times* (London), December 5, 1999, p. 11.

140. A. Relman, quoted in "Payer failure," *AAPS (Association of American Physicians and Surgeons) News,* 56: 1 (March), 2000.

141. M. Angell, "Patients' rights bills and other futile gestures" (Editorial), *New England Journal of Medicine,* 342: 1663–1664 (June 1), 2000, p. 1664.

142. H. Pardes, "Academic medicine: Perilous condition" (Letters), *New York Times,* June 24, 2000, Internet edition, emphasis added.

143. Quoted in J. Fallows, "The political scientist: Harold Varmus has ambitious plans for the future of medicine," *New Yorker,* June 7, 1999, pp. 66–75, p. 68.

144. R. Cobden, in *Russia* [1836], quoted in *Ideas on Liberty,* February 2000, back cover.

145. T. S. Szasz, *Ceremonial Chemistry.*

146. See, for example, D. McCloskey, *Crossing.*

147. R. Hayes and E. LeBrun, "Public health surveillance for firearm injuries," *JAMA,* 282: 429–430 (August 4), 1999.

148. A. Gore, "Gore sets goal for a cancer-free America," www.algore2000. com/briefingroom/releases/pr_06t01_GA_1.html; quoted in T. Dalrymple, "War against cancer won't be won soon," *Wall Street Journal,* June 11, 2000, p. A30.

149. P. Brimelow, "The lawyer spigot," *Forbes,* September 20, 1999, p. 150.

150. A. Ferguson, "What politicians can't do," *Time,* May 3, 1999, p. 52.

EPILOGUE

1. A. B. Casares, "Plans for an escape to Carmelo," *New York Review of Books,* April 10, 1986, p. 7.

2. F. Bastiat, *Selected Essays on Political Economy,* p. 13, emphasis added.

3. Quoted in R. Higgs, "Lock 'em up!" *The Independent Review,* 4: 309–313 (Fall), 1999, p. 313.

4. T. S. Szasz, "Patriotic poisoners," *Humanist,* 36: 5–7 (November–December), 1976. See also J. D. Moreno, *Undue Risk;* E. Welsome, *The Plutonium Files;* and Associated Press, "Test drugs OK'd for mentally ill," *New York Times,* November 29, 1999, Internet edition.

5. W. B. Schwartz, *Life without Disease.*

6. Paper delivered at the Seventh Annual Euthanasia Conference, New York, December 1974; quoted in J. Boyle and J. Morris, "The crisis in medicine: Models, myth, and metaphors," *Reflections,* 16: 14–27, 1981, pp. 25–26.

7. Front cover. S. S. Hall, "The recycled generation," *New York Times Magazine,* January 30, 2000, pp. 30 ff.

8. W. Safire, "Why die?," *New York Times,* January 1, 2000, Internet edition.

9. Associated Press, "Some criticism of Reeve walking ad," *New York Times,* January 31, 2000. Internet edition.

10. T. S. Szasz, *The Theology of Medicine.*

11. J. W. von Goethe, "Letter to Charlotte von Stein" (June 8, 1787), in *Gedenkausgabe,* 11: 362. My translation.

12. J. Romains, *Knock,* p. 35.

SELECTED BIBLIOGRAPHY

References to articles, reports, and other items appearing in journals, magazines, newspapers, and pamphlets are fully identified in the Notes. Books cited in the Notes only by author and title are identified more fully below.

Ackerknecht, E. H. *Rudolf Virchow: Doctor, Statesman, Anthropologist.* Madison University of Wisconsin Press, 1953.

Adler, M. J. *What Man Has Made of Man: A Study of the Consequences of Platonism and Positivism in Psychology.* New York: Frederick Ungar, 1937.

Allan, K., and Burridge, K. *Euphemism and Dysphemism: Language Used as Shield and Weapon.* New York: Oxford University Press, 1991.

American Medical Association. *Guides to the Evaluation of Permanent Impairment.* 4th edition. Chicago: American Medical Association, 1993.

American Psychiatric Association. *Diagnostic and Statistical Manual of Mental Disorders—III.* 3rd ed. Washington, DC: American Psychiatric Association, 1980.

American Psychiatric Association. *Diagnostic and Statistical Manual of Mental Disorders—IV.* 4th ed. Washington, DC: American Psychiatric Association, 1994.

American Psychiatric Association. *Diagnostic and Statistical Manual of Mental Disorders of the American Psychiatric Association (DSM-III-R).* Third Edition—Revised. Washington, DC: American Psychiatric Association, 1987.

American Psychiatric Association. *DSM-IV Options Book: Work in Progress.* Washington, DC: American Psychiatric Association, 1991.

Selected Bibliography

Annas, G. J. *Some Choice: Law, Medicine, and the Market*. New York: Oxford University Press, 1998.

Arieti, S. *Interpretation of Schizophrenia*. 2nd ed. New York: Basic Books, 1974.

Aristotle. *The Basic Works of Aristotle*. Edited by Richard McKeon. New York: Random House, 1941.

Arney, W. R., and Bergen, B. J. *Medicine and the Management of Living: Taming the Last Great Beast*. Chicago: University of Chicago Press, 1984.

Aronowitz, R. A. *Making Sense of Illness: Science, Society, and Disease*. Cambridge: Cambridge University Press, 1998.

Auden, W. H. *The Dyer's Hand, and Other Essays* [1962]. New York: Vintage, 1968.

Balázs, E. *Chinese Civilization and Bureaucracy: Variations on a Theme*. Translated by H. M. Wright. New Haven: Yale University Press, 1964.

Barker, P. *Regeneration*. New York: Penguin/Plume, 1993.

Bartlett, J. *Familiar Quotations*. 12th ed. Edited by Christopher Morley. Boston: Little, Brown & Co., 1951.

Bartlett, J. *Familiar Quotations*. 16th ed. Edited by Justin Kaplan. Boston: Little, Brown & Co., 1992.

Bastiat, F. *Selected Essays on Political Economy*. Edited by George B. De Huszar. Irvington-on-Hudson, NY: Foundation for Economic Education, 1964.

Beauchamp, D. E. *Health Care Reform and the Battle for the Body Politic*. Philadelphia: Temple University Press, 1996.

Beauchamp, D. E. *The Health of the Republic: Epidemics, Medicine, and Moralism as Challenges to Democracy*. Philadelphia: Temple University Press, 1988.

Beauchamp, D. E., and Steinbock, B., eds. *New Ethics for the Public's Health*. New York: Oxford University Press, 1999.

Beauchamp, T. L., and Walters, L., eds. *Contemporary Issues in Bioethics*. Encino, CA: Dickenson Publishing Co., 1978.

Bennett, J. C., and Plum, F., eds. *Cecil Textbook of Medicine*. 10th ed. 3 vols. Philadelphia: W. B. Saunders, 1995.

Bennett, J. T., and DiLorenzo, T. J. *The Food and Drink Police: America's Nannies, Busybodies, and Petty Tyrants*. New Brunswick, NJ: Transaction, 1999.

Bidinotto, R. J. ed. *Criminal Justice? The Legal System versus Individual Responsibility*. Irvington-on-Hudson, NY: Foundation for Economic Education, 1996.

Binger, C. *Revolutionary Doctor: Benjamin Rush, 1746–1813*. New York: Norton, 1966.

Bleuler, E. *Dementia Praecox or the Group of Schizophrenias* [1911]. Translated by Joseph Zinkin. New York: International Universities Press, 1950.

Bleuler, E. *A Textbook of Psychiatry* [1924]. Translated by A. A. Brill. New York: Macmillan, 1944.

Bleuler, M. *The Schizophrenic Disorders: Long-Term Patient and Family Studies* [1972]. Translated by Siegfried M. Clemens. New Haven: Yale University Press, 1978.

Bloch, S., and Chodoff, P., eds. *Psychiatric Ethics*. 2nd ed. Oxford: Oxford University Press, 1991.

Selected Bibliography

Bloch, S., Chodoff, P., and Green, S. A., eds. *Psychiatric Ethics.* 3rd ed. Oxford: Oxford University Press, 1999.

Bloch, S., and Reddaway, P. *Psychiatric Terror: How Soviet Psychiatry Is Used to Suppress Dissent.* New York: Basic Books, 1977.

Borkin, J. *The Crime and Punishment of I. G. Farben* [1978]. New York: Barnes & Noble, 1997.

Bourne, R. *The Radical Will: Selected Writings, 1911–1918.* New York: Urizen Books, 1977.

Bovard, J. *Freedom in Chains: The Rise of the State and the Demise of the Citizen.* New York: St. Martin's Press, 1999.

Boyd, B. A. *Rudolf Virchow: The Scientist as Citizen.* New York: Garland Publishing, 1991.

Braslow, J. *Mental Ills and Bodily Cures: Psychiatric Treatment in the First Half of the Twentieth Century.* Berkeley: University of California Press, 1997.

Buchanan, J. M. *The Limits of Liberty: Between Anarchy and Leviathan.* Chicago: University of Chicago Press, 1975.

Burke, E. *The Philosophy of Edmund Burke: A Selection from His Speeches and Writings.* Edited with an Introduction by Louis I. Bredvold and Ralph G. Ross. Ann Arbor: University of Michigan Press, 1961.

Canguilhem, G. *On the Normal and the Pathological.* Boston: D. Reidel, 1978.

Caplan, A. L., Engelhardt, H. T., Jr., and McCartney, J. J., eds. *Concepts of Health and Disease: Interdisciplinary Perspectives.* Reading, MA: Addison-Wesley Publishing Company, 1981.

Carlyle, T. *Sartor Resartus.* New York: Home Book Co., 1890.

Cassell, E. J. *The Nature of Suffering and the Goals of Medicine.* New York: Oxford University Press, 1991.

Chadwick, O. *Professor Lord Acton: The Regius Chair of Modern History at Cambridge, 1895–1902.* Grand Rapids, MI: Acton Institute, 1995.

Chesterton, G. K. *Orthodoxy.* London: John Lane, 1909.

Chesterton, G. K. *The Quotable Chesterton: A Topical Compilation of the Wit, Wisdom and Satire of G. K. Chesterton.* Edited by George J. Marlin, Richard P. Rabatin, and John L. Swan. San Francisco: Ignatius Press, 1986.

Coiera, E. *Guide to Medical Informatics, the Internet and Telemedicine.* London: Chapman & Hall Medical, 1997.

Cotran, R. S., Kumar, V., Collins, T., and Robbins, S. L., eds. *Robbins Pathologic Basis of Disease.* 6th ed. Philadelphia: W. B. Saunders, 1999.

Cotran, R. S., Kumar, V., Robbins, S. L., and Schoen, F. J., eds. *Robbins Pathologic Basis of Disease.* 5th ed. Philadelphia: W. B. Saunders, 1994.

Creveld, M. van. *The Rise and Decline of the State.* Cambridge: Cambridge University Press, 1999.

Critchley, M., ed. *Butterworth's Medical Dictionary.* 2nd ed. London: Butterworths, 1978.

Culver, C. M., and Gert, B. *Philosophy in Medicine: Conceptual and Ethical Issues in Medicine and Psychiatry.* New York: Oxford University Press, 1982.

Selected Bibliography

Damjanov, I., and Linder, J., eds. *Anderson's Pathology*. 10th ed. St. Louis: Mosby, 1996.

Daniels, N. *Just Health Care*. Cambridge: Cambridge University Press, 1985.

Deutsch, A. *The Mentally Ill in America: A History of Their Care and Treatment from Colonial Times* (1937). 2nd ed. New York: Columbia University Press, 1949.

Dixon, R. *The Baumgarten Corruption: From Sense to Nonsense in Art and Philosophy*. London: Pluto Press, 1995.

Dubos, R. J. *Louis Pasteur: Free Lance of Science*. Boston: Little, Brown and Company, 1950.

Duster, T. *Backdoor to Eugenics*. New York: Routledge, 1990.

Edwards, R. B., and Graber, G. C., eds. *Bioethics*. New York: Harcourt Brace Jovanovich, 1988.

Encyclopaedia Britannica. Chicago: Encyclopaedia Britannica, 1973.

Encyclopedia of the Social Sciences, International. Edited by David L. Sils. New York: Macmillan and Free Press, 1968.

Engelhardt, H. T., Jr., and Spicker, S. F., eds. *Evaluation and Explanation in the Biomedical Sciences*. Dordrecht, Neth.: D. Reidel, 1975.

Fabrega, H., Jr. *Evolution of Sickness and Healing*. Berkeley: University of California Press, 1997.

Fadiman, A. *The Spirit Catches You and You Fall Down: A Hmong Child, Her American Doctors, & the Collision of Two Cultures*. New York: Farrar, Straus & Giroux, 1997.

Feinstein, A. R. *Clinical Judgment*. Baltimore: Williams & Wilkins, 1967.

Feldman, M., Ford, C. C., and Reinhold, T. *Patient or Pretender: Inside the Strange World of Factitious Disorders*. John Wiley & Sons, 1994.

Fetter, R. B., ed. *DRGs, Their Design and Development*. Ann Arbor, MI: Health Administration Press, 1991.

Feynman, R. P. *"What Do You Care What Other People Think?": Further Adventures of a Curious Character*. New York: Bantam Books, 1989.

Flack, W. F., Jr., Miller, D. R., and Wiener, M., eds. *What is Schizophrenia?* New York: Springer Verlag, 1991.

Flynn, J. T. *The Roosevelt Myth* [1948]. San Francisco: Fox & Wilkes, 1998.

Foundation for Economic Education. *Politicized Medicine*. Irvington-on-Hudson, NY: Foundation for Economic Education, 1993.

Frank, L. R., ed. *Random House Webster's Quotationary*. New York: Random House, 1999.

Freud, S. *The Complete Letters of Sigmund Freud to Wilhelm Fliess, 1887–1904*. Translated and edited by Jeffrey Moussaieff Masson. Cambridge: Belknap Press/Harvard University Press, 1985.

Freud, S. *The Standard Edition of the Complete Psychological Works of Sigmund Freud*. Translated by James Strachey. 24 vols. London: Hogarth Press, 1953–1974. Cited as *SE*.

Friedlander, H. *The Origins of Nazi Genocide: From Euthanasia to the Final Solution.* Chapel Hill: University of North Carolina Press, 1995.

Fulford, K. W. M. *Moral Theory and Medical Practice.* Cambridge: Cambridge University Press, 1989.

Garrison, F. H. *An Introduction to the History of Medicine: With Medical Chronology, Suggestions for Study and Bibliographic Data* (1913). 4th ed. Philadelphia: W. B. Saunders, 1929.

Gaylin, W., and Jennings, B. *The Perversion of Autonomy: The Proper Uses of Coercion and Constraints in a Liberal Society.* New York: Free Press, 1996.

Gert, B., Culver, C. M., and Clouser, K. D. *Bioethics: A Return to Fundamentals.* New York: Oxford University Press, 1977.

Gilman, S. L. *Sexuality: An Illustrated History.* New York: John Wiley & Sons, 1989.

Gilman, S. L., King, H., Porter, R., Rousseau, G. S., and Showalter, E. *Hysteria beyond Freud.* Berkeley: University of California Press, 1993.

Gleick, J. *Genius: The Life and Science of Richard Feynman.* New York: Pantheon, 1992.

Goodwin, D. W., and Guze, S. B. *Psychiatric Diagnosis.* 5th ed. New York: Oxford University Press, 1996.

Goodwin, F. K., and Jamison, K. R. *Manic-Depressive Illness.* New York: Oxford University Press, 1990.

Gregory, I. *Fundamentals of Psychiatry.* Philadelphia: W. B. Saunders, 1968, p. 32.

Gross, P. R., Levitt, N., and Lewis, M. W. *The Flight from Science and Reason.* New York: New York Academy of Sciences, 1996. (*Annals of the New York Academy of Sciences*, vol. 775.)

Grun, B. *The Timetables of History: A Horizontal Linkage of People and Events.* New, updated edition. New York: Touchstone/Simon & Schuster, 1982.

Guterman, N. *The Anchor Book of Latin Quotations*, compiled by Norbert Guterman. New York: Doubleday, 1966.

Guze, S. B. *Why Psychiatry Is a Branch of Medicine.* New York: Oxford University Press, 1992.

Haack, S. *Manifesto of a Passionate Moderate: Unfashionable Essays.* Chicago: University of Chicago Press, 1998.

Harrison, T. R., et al., eds. *Principles of Internal Medicine.* 9th ed. Philadelphia: Blakiston, 1950.

Haveman, R. H., Halberstadt, V., and Burkhauser, R. V. *Public Policy toward Disabled Workers: Cross-National Analyses of Economic Impacts.* Ithaca, NY: Cornell University Press, 1984.

Hayek, F. A. *The Counter-Revolution of Science: Studies in the Abuse of Reason.* New York: Free Press, 1955.

Higgs, R. *Crisis and Leviathan: Critical Episodes in the Growth of American Government.* New York: Oxford University Press, 1987.

Himmelfarb, G. *The Idea of Poverty: England in the Early Industrial Age.* New York: Random House, 1983.

Selected Bibliography

Hunter, R., and Macalpine, I. *Psychiatry for the Poor, 1851. Colney Hatch Asylum, Friern Hospital, 1973: A Medical and Social History.* London: Dawson, 1974.

Hunter, R., and Macalpine, I., eds. *Three Hundred Years of Psychiatry, 1535–1860: A History Presented in Selected English Texts.* London: Oxford University Press, 1963.

Ifrah, G. *The Universal History of Numbers: From Prehistory to the Invention of the Computer* [1994]. New York: Wiley, 2000.

Illich, I. *Medical Nemesis: The Expropriation of Health.* New York: Pantheon, 1976.

Jarausch, K. H. *The Unfree Professions: German Lawyers, Teachers, and Engineers, 1900–1950.* New York: Oxford University Press, 1950.

Jaspers, K. *General Psychopathology* [1913, 1946]. 7th ed. Chicago: University of Chicago Press, 1963.

Johnson, S. *Johnson's Dictionary: A Modern Selection* [1755]. Edited by E. L. McAdam, Jr. and George Milne. New York: Pantheon, 1963.

Jones, M., ed. *Fake? The Art of Deception.* Berkeley: University of California Press, 1990.

Kaplan, H. I., and Saddock, B. J., eds. *Comprehensive Textbook of Psychiatry/VI.* 6th ed. 2 vols.; Baltimore: Williams & Wilkins, 1995.

Kershaw, I. *Hitler: 1889–1936: Hubris.* New York: Norton, 1999.

Kessler, H. H. *Disability: Determination and Evaluation.* Philadelphia: Lea & Febiger, 1970.

King, L. *The Growth of Medical Thought.* Chicago: University of Chicago Press, 1963.

King, S. H. *Perceptions of Illness and Medical Practice.* New York: Russell Sage, 1962.

Kirk, S. A., and Kutchins, H. *The Selling of DSM: The Rhetoric of Science in Psychiatry.* New York: Aldine de Gruyter, 1992.

Klein, D. F., and Wender, P. H. *Understanding Depression: A Complete Guide to Its Diagnosis and Treatment.* New York: Oxford University Press, 1993.

Kleinman, A. *The Illness Narratives: Suffering, Healing, and the Human Condition.* New York: Basic Books, 1988.

Koch, A. *Madison's "Advice to My Country."* Princeton: Princeton University Press, 1966.

Kosinski, J. *The Painted Bird.* Boston: Houghton Mifflin, 1965.

Kraepelin, E. *Einführung in die psychiatrische Klinik.* Leipzig: Johann Ambrosius Barth, 1901.

Kraepelin, E. *Lectures on Clinical Psychiatry* [1901]. New York: Hafner, 1968.

Krafft-Ebing, R. *Psychopathia Sexualis, with Special Reference to the Antipathic Sexual Instinct: A Medico-Forensic Study* [1886/1906]. Authorized English adaptation of the twelfth German edition by F. J. Rebman. Revised edition. Brooklyn, NY: Physicians and Surgeons Book Company, 1931.

Lawson, N. *The Retreat of the State.* Norwich, CT: Canterbury Press, 2000.

Levin, A. V., and Sheridan, M. S. *Münchausen Syndrome: Issues in Diagnosis and Treatment.* New York: Lexington Books, 1995.

Selected Bibliography

Lewis, C. S. *The Abolition of Man*. New York: Macmillan, 1947.

Lewis, C. S. *The Business of Heaven: Daily Readings from C. S. Lewis*. Edited with a preface by Walter Hooper. New York: Harcourt Brace Jovanovich, 1984.

Lewis, C. S. *God in the Dock: Essays on Theology and Ethics*. Edited by Walter Hooper. Grand Rapids, MI: William B. Eerdmans, 1970.

Lowi, T. J. *The End of Liberalism: Ideology, Policy, and the Crisis of Public Authority*. New York: Norton, 1969.

Lush, B., ed. *Concepts of Medicine: A Collection of Essays on Aspects of Medicine*. New York: Pergamon, 1961.

Lynch, M. J., and Raphael, S. S. *Medicine and the State*. Oak Brook, IL: Association of American Physicians and Surgeons, 1973.

Mackay, C. *Extraordinary Popular Delusions and the Madness of Crowds* [1841, 1852]. New York: Noonday Press, 1962.

Magner, L. N. *A History of Medicine*. New York: Marcel Dekker, 1992.

Maine, H. S. *Ancient Law: Its Connection with the Early History of Society, and Its Relation to Modern Ideas* [1846]. Tucson: University of Arizona Press, 1986.

Mann, T. *Confessions of Felix Krull, Confidence Man* [1954]. Translated by Denver Lindley. New York: Signet/New American Library, 1957.

Marks, J. *The Search for the "Manchurian Candidate": The CIA and Mind Control*. New York: Times Books, 1979.

McCloskey, D. *Crossing: A Memoir*. Chicago: University of Chicago Press, 1999.

McKinney's Consolidated Laws of New York. St. Paul, MN: West Publishing Company, 1993.

Meiklejohn, A. *Political Freedom: The Constitutional Powers of the People*. New York: Harper & Brothers, 1960.

Menninger, K. *The Crime of Punishment*. New York: Viking, 1968.

Menninger, K. *The Vital Balance: The Life Process in Mental Health and Illness*. New York: Viking, 1963.

Mettler, C. C., and Mettler, F. A. *History of Medicine: A Correlative Text, Arranged According to Subjects*. Philadelphia: Blakiston, 1947.

Meynert, T. *Psychiatry: Clinical Treatise on Diseases of the Forebrain* [1884]. Translated by B. Sachs. New York: G. P. Putnam's Sons, 1885.

Micale, M. S., and Porter, R., eds. *Discovering the History of Psychiatry*. New York: Oxford University Press, 1994.

Mill, J. S. *On Liberty* [1859]. Chicago: Regnery, 1955.

Mises, L. von. *Human Action: A Treatise on Economics*. New Haven: Yale University Press, 1949.

Mises, L. von. *Omnipotent Government: The Rise of the Total State and Total War* [1944]. Spring Mills, PA: Libertarian Press, 1985.

Mises, L. von. *Socialism: An Economic and Sociological Analysis* [1922]. Translated by J. Kahane. Indianapolis: Liberty Fund, 1981.

Mises, L. von. *The Theory of Money and Credit* [1912]. Translated by H. E. Bateson. Indianapolis: LibertyClassics, 1980.

Selected Bibliography

Molière. *The Misanthrope and Other Plays.* Translated by J. Wood. Baltimore: Penguin, 1959.

Moore, M. S. *Law and Psychiatry: Rethinking the Relationship.* New York: Cambridge University Press, 1984.

Moreno, J. D. *Undue Risk: Secret State Experiments on Humans.* New York: W. H. Freeman, 1999.

Morris, D. B. *Illness and Culture in the Postmodern Age.* Berkeley: University of California Press, 1998.

Moscovit, A. *Our Choice and History.* Translated by Isabel Heaman. New York: Philosophical Library, 1985.

Muller-Hill, B. *Murderous Science.* New York: Oxford University Press, 1988.

Munthe, A. *The Story of San Michele* [1929]. New York: Dutton, 1957.

Murray, G. *Five Stages of Greek Religion.* Garden City, NY: Doubleday Anchor, 1955.

Nolan, J. L., Jr. *The Therapeutic State: Justifying Government at Century's End.* New York: New York University Press, 1998.

Osler, W. *Aequanimitas: With Other Addresses to Medical Students, Nurses and Practitioners of Medicine.* 3rd ed. Philadelphia: Blakiston, 1943.

Oxford Dictionary of Quotations, The. 4th ed. Edited by Angela Partington. New York: Oxford University Press, 1992.

Paarlberg, D. *An Analysis and History of Inflation.* Westport, CT: Praeger, 1993.

Plato. *Republic.* In Plato, *The Collected Dialogues of Plato, Including the Letters.* Edited by Edith Hamilton and Huntington Cairns. Princeton: Princeton University Press, 1961.

Polanyi, M. *Knowing and Being: Essays by Michael Polanyi.* Edited by Marjorie Grene. Chicago: University of Chicago Press, 1969.

Polanyi, M. *Personal Knowledge: Towards a Post-Critical Philosophy.* Chicago: University of Chicago Press, 1958.

Porter, B. D. *War and the Rise of the State: The Military Foundations of Modern Politics.* New York: Free Press, 1994.

Poynter, F. N. L., ed. *Medicine and Science in the 1860s.* London: Wellcome Institute of the History of Medicine, 1968.

Proctor, R. N. *The Nazi War on Cancer.* Princeton: Princeton University Press, 1999.

Ratey, J. J., and Johnson, C. *Shadow Syndromes.* New York: Pantheon, 1997.

Rather, L. J., ed. *Disease, Life, and Man: Selected Essays by Rudolf Virchow.* Stanford: Stanford University Press, 1958.

Reiser, S. J. *Medicine and the Reign of Technology.* Cambridge: Cambridge University Press, 1978.

Reno, V., Mashaw, J. L., and Gradison, B., eds. *Disability: Challenges for Social Insurance, Health Care Financing and Labor Market Policy.* Washington, DC: National Academy of Social Insurance, 1997.

Revel, J.-F. *The Totalitarian Temptation.* Translated by David Hapgood. Garden City, NY: Doubleday, 1977.

Reznek, L. *Evil or Ill?: Justifying the Insanity Defense.* London: Routledge, 1997.

Reznek, L. *The Nature of Disease.* London: Routledge, 1987.

Reznek, L. *The Philosophical Defence of Psychiatry.* London: Routledge, 1991.

Riese, W. *The Conception of Disease: Its History, Its Versions, and Its Nature.* New York: Philosophical Library, 1953.

Ritvo, H. *The Platypus and the Mermaid, and Other Figments of the Classifying Imagination.* Cambridge: Harvard University Press, 1997.

Robbins, S. L. *Pathologic Basis of Disease.* 1st ed. Philadelphia: W. B. Saunders, 1974.

Robitscher, J. *The Powers of Psychiatry.* Boston: Houghton Mifflin, 1980.

Romains, J. *Knock [Knock, ou le Triomphe de la Médecine, 1923].* Translated by James B. Gidney. Great Neck, NY: Barron Educational Series, 1962.

Rousseau, G. S., ed. *The Languages of Psyche: Mind and Body in Enlightenment Thought.* Berkeley: University of California Press, 1990.

Rubin, E., and Farber, J. L. *Pathology.* Philadelphia: Lippincott, 1994.

Rycroft, C. *Anxiety and Neurosis.* Baltimore: Penguin, 1968.

Rycroft, R. *A Critical Dictionary of Psychoanalysis.* 2nd ed. Harmondsworth: Penguin, 1995.

Sadler, J. Z., Wigging, O. P., and Schwartz, M.A., eds. *Philosophical Perspectives on Psychiatric Diagnostic Classification.* Baltimore: Johns Hopkins University Press, 1994.

Schaler, J. A. *Addiction Is a Choice.* Chicago: Open Court, 2000.

Schmukler, N., and Marcus, E., eds. *Inflation Through the Ages: Economic, Social, Psychological, and Historical Aspects.* New York: Brooklyn College Press/Columbia University Press, 1983.

Schreber, D. *Memoirs of My Nervous Illness* [1903]. Translated by Ida Macalpine and Richard Hunter. London: William Dawson & Sons, 1955.

Schwartz, W. B. *Life without Disease: The Pursuit of Medical Utopia.* Berkeley: University of California Press, 1998.

Sedgwick, P. *Psychopolitics.* New York: Harper & Row, 1982.

Sharkey, J. *Bedlam: Greed, Profiteering, and Fraud in a Mental Health System Gone Crazy.* New York: St. Martin's Press, 1994.

Simon, J. *Hoodwinking the Nation.* New Brunswick, NJ: Transaction Publishers, 1999.

Singer, P. *Practical Ethics.* 2nd ed. Cambridge: Cambridge University Press, 1993.

Singer, P. *Rethinking Life and Death: The Collapse of Our Traditional Ethics.* New York: St. Martin's Press, 1994.

Sloan, J. P. *Jerzy Kosinski: A Biography.* New York: Dutton, 1996.

Snell, B. *The Discovery of the Mind: The Greek Origins of European Thought* (1948). Translated by T. G. Rosenmeyer. New York: Harper Torchbook, 1960.

Stevenson, L. G., ed. *A Celebration of Medical History: The Fiftieth Anniversary of the Johns Hopkins Institute of the History of Medicine and the Welch Medical Library.* Baltimore: The Johns Hopkins University Press, 1982.

Strange, S. *The Retreat of the State: The Diffusion of Power in the World Economy.* Cambridge: Cambridge University Press, 1996.

Swann, D. *The Retreat of the State: Deregulation and Privatization in the UK and US.* Ann Arbor: University of Michigan Press, 1998.

Szasz, T. S. *Anti-Freud: Karl Kraus's Criticism of Psychoanalysis and Psychiatry* [1976]. Syracuse: Syracuse University Press, 1990.

Szasz, T. S. *Ceremonial Chemistry: The Ritual Persecution of Drugs, Addicts, and Pushers* [1976]. Revised edition. Holmes Beach, FL: Learning Publications, 1985.

Szasz, T. S. *Cruel Compassion: The Psychiatric Control of Society's Unwanted* [1994]. Syracuse: Syracuse University Press, 1998.

Szasz, T. S. *The Ethics of Psychoanalysis: The Theory and Method of Autonomous Psychotherapy* [1965]. With a new preface. Syracuse: Syracuse University Press, 1988.

Szasz, T. S. *Fatal Freedom: The Ethics and Politics of Suicide.* Westport, CT: Praeger, 1999.

Szasz, T. S. *Insanity: The Idea and Its Consequences* [1987]. Syracuse: Syracuse University Press, 1997.

Szasz, T. S. *Law, Liberty, and Psychiatry: An Inquiry into the Social Uses of Mental Health Practices* [1963]. Syracuse: Syracuse University Press, 1989.

Szasz, T. S. *A Lexicon of Lunacy: Metaphoric Malady, Moral Responsibility, and Psychiatry.* New Brunswick, NJ: Transaction Publishers, 1993.

Szasz, T. S. *The Manufacture of Madness: A Comparative Study of the Inquisition and the Mental Health Movement* [1970]. With a new preface. Syracuse: Syracuse University Press, 1997.

Szasz, T. S. *The Meaning of Mind: Language, Morality, and Neuroscience.* New York: Praeger, 1996.

Szasz, T. S. *The Myth of Mental Illness: Foundations of a Theory of Personal Conduct* [1961]. Revised edition. New York: HarperCollins, 1974.

Szasz, T. S. *The Myth of Psychotherapy: Mental Healing as Religion, Rhetoric, and Repression* [1978]. Syracuse: Syracuse University Press, 1988.

Szasz, T. S. *Our Right to Drugs: The Case for a Free Market.* Westport, CT: Praeger, 1992.

Szasz, T. S. *Pain and Pleasure: A Study of Bodily Feelings* [1957]. Second expanded edition [1975]. Syracuse: Syracuse University Press, 1988.

Szasz, T. S. *Psychiatric Justice* [1965]. With a new preface. Syracuse: Syracuse University Press, 1988.

Szasz, T. S. *Psychiatric Slavery: When Confinement and Coercion Masquerade as Cure* [1977]. Syracuse: Syracuse University Press, 1989.

Szasz, T. S. *The Second Sin.* Garden City, NY: Doubleday Anchor, 1973.

Szasz, T. S. *Sex by Prescription* [1980]. Syracuse: Syracuse University Press, 1990.

Szasz, T. S. *The Theology of Medicine: The Political-Philosophical Foundations of Medical Ethics* [1977]. With a new preface. Syracuse: Syracuse University Press, 1988.

Szasz, T. S. *The Therapeutic State: Psychiatry in the Mirror of Current Events*. Buffalo: Prometheus Books, 1984.

Szasz, T. S. *The Untamed Tongue: A Dissenting Dictionary*. LaSalle, IL: Open Court, 1990.

Szasz, T. S., ed. *The Age of Madness: A History of Involuntary Mental Hospitalization Presented in Selected Texts*. Garden City, NY: Doubleday Anchor, 1973.

Thagard, P. *How Scientists Explain Disease*. Princeton: Princeton University Press, 1999.

Thomas, K. *Religion and the Decline of Magic*. London: Weidenfeld & Nicholson, 1971.

Tocqueville, A. de. *Democracy in America* [1835–1840]. Edited by Phillips Bradley. 2 vols. New York: Vintage, 1945.

Todorov, T. *Mikhail Bakhtin: The Dialogical Principle* [1981]. Translated by Wlad Godzich. Minneapolis: University of Minnesota Press, 1984.

Traupman, J. C. *The New College Latin and English Dictionary*. New York: Bantam, 1966.

U.S. Department of Commerce. *Statistical Abstracts of the United States, 1998*. 118th edition. Washington, DC: U.S. Census Bureau, October 1998.

U.S. Department of Health and Human Services. *Health, United States, 1998*. Washington, DC: DHHS publication number (PHS) 98–1232, 1998.

Veith, I. *The Yellow Emperor's Classic of Internal Medicine*. Berkeley: University of California Press, 1966.

Webb, S., and Webb, B. *The State and the Doctor*. London: Longmans, Green and Co., 1910.

Weindling, P. *Health, Race and German Politics between National Unification and Nazism, 1870–1945*. Cambridge: Cambridge University Press, 1989.

Welsome, E. *The Plutonium Files: America's Secret Medical Experiments in the Cold War*. New York: Dial Press, 1999.

Wilbur, G. B., and Muensterberger, W., eds. *Psychoanalysis and Culture*. New York: International Universities Press, 1951.

Wilkomirski, B. *Fragments: Memories of a Wartime Childhood*. Translated by Carol Brown Janeway. New York: Schocken, 1966.

Woodward, K. L. *Making Saints: How the Catholic Church Determines Who Becomes a Saint, Who Doesn't, and Why*. New York: Simon & Schuster, 1990.

Woolf, V. *On Being Ill*. London: Hogarth Press, 1930.

World Almanac and Book of Facts, 1999. Mahwah, NJ: World Almanac Books, 1999.

Zagorin, P. *Ways of Lying: Dissimulation, Persecution, and Conformity in Early Modern Europe*. Cambridge: Harvard University Press, 1990.

Zilboorg, G. *A History of Medical Psychology*. In collaboration with G. W. Henry. New York: Norton, 1941.

INDEX

Index

About the Author

THOMAS SZASZ is Professor of Psychiatry Emeritus, State University of New York Upstate Medical University, Syracuse, New York. He is the author of *Our Right to Drugs* (Praeger, 1992), *The Meaning of Mind* (Praeger, 1996), and *Fatal Freedom* (Praeger, 1999).